130 Kidney Disease Juice and Meal Recipes:

Give Your Body What It Needs to Recover Fast and Naturally

By

Joe Correa CSN

COPYRIGHT

This publication is designed to provide accurate and authoritative information in regard to the subject matter covered. It is sold with the understanding that neither the author nor the publisher is engaged in rendering medical advice. If medical advice or assistance is needed, consult with a doctor. This book is considered a guide and should not be used in any way detrimental to your health. Consult with a physician before starting this nutritional plan to make sure it's right for you.

ACKNOWLEDGEMENTS

This book is dedicated to my friends and family that have had mild or serious illnesses so that you may find a solution and make the necessary changes in your life.

130 Kidney Disease Juice and Meal Recipes:

Give Your Body What It Needs to Recover Fast and Naturally

By

Joe Correa CSN

CONTENTS

ABOUT THE AUTHOR

After years of Research, I honestly believe in the positive effects that proper nutrition can have over the body and mind. My knowledge and experience has helped me live healthier throughout the years and which I have shared with family and friends. The more you know about eating and drinking healthier, the sooner you will want to change your life and eating habits.

Nutrition is a key part in the process of being healthy and living longer so get started today. The first step is the most important and the most significant.

INTRODUCTION

130 Kidney Disease Juice and Meal Recipes: Give Your Body What It Needs to Recover Fast and Naturally

By Joe Correa CSN

Kidney disease is defined as any form of abnormality in these organs. These abnormalities prevent normal kidney function and lead to some serious medical conditions, mainly waste products are kept inside your body. Without a proper treatment, kidney disease can lead to complete kidney failure and a life-threatening condition.

The main causes of kidney disease are diabetes, high blood pressure, urinary tract infections, overuse of different drugs, inherited kidney disease, and of course an unhealthy diet based on highly processed foods full of different chemicals. In order to keep your kidneys healthy and prevent complications, you need to learn how to recognize the first symptoms related to kidney disease. These symptoms include poor sleep, swelling in your ankles, vomiting, overall weakness and lack of energy, shortness of breath, and urination problems. All of these symptoms should be examined by your physician to determine their cause.

Just like every other medical condition, kidney disease is closely related to a poor diet and an unhealthy lifestyle. Researchers have discovered numerous links between inflammation and some foods that are able to prevent chronic and degenerative conditions. Foods like bell peppers, cabbage, cauliflower, garlic, apples, cranberries, blueberries, raspberries, cherries, and grapes are rich in antioxidants that are able to neutralize free radicals and protect the body. These foods are the basis of a healthy, kidney-friendly diet and should be included in your meals and juices every day.

The juice and meal récipes in this book will help you to treat and overcome kidney disease and live a healthier life.

130 KIDNEY DISEASE JUICE AND MEAL RECIPES: GIVE YOUR BODY WHAT IT NEEDS TO RECOVER FAST AND NATURALLY

MEALS

1.   Lactose free milk with coffee, whole meal bread with cheese and pear

Ingredients:

- 1 cup of lactose free milk

- 2 spoons of coffee

- 2 slices of whole meal bread

- 2 slices of cheese

- 1 pear

Procedure: One cup of lactose free milk with coffee, two slices of whole meal bread with cheese and one pear.

Nutritional facts: Energy 254 kcal, proteins 15.4 g, total fat 4.2 g, cholesterol 5.6 mg, carbohydrates 39.7 g, fiber 6.5 g and sodium 486 mg.

2.   Peach and papaya juice, yogurt with apple and oats

Ingredients:

- 1/2 cup of peach
- 1/2 cup of papaya
- 1/2 cup of water
- 125 g of lactose free yogurt
- 3 spoons of instant oats
- 1 apple

Procedure: In the blender, mix half cup of peach and papaya with half cup of water. Mix the lactose free yogurt (125 g) with three spoons of instant oats and an apple in squares.

Nutritional facts: Energy 255 kcal, protein 14.9 g, total fat 2.2 g, cholesterol 2.8 mg, carbohydrates 37.9 g, fiber 4.1 g and sodium 12.3 mg.

3. Filled tomatoes with tuna

Ingredients:

- 6 tomatoes
- 2 cups of boiled corn
- 1/2 cup of onion cut in squares
- 1/2 cup of olive oil
- 1 can of tuna
- parsley
- salt and pepper
- lettuce

Procedure: Wash the tomatoes and take out the top, make a hole and take out what is inside with a spoon. Cut the seeds from inside the tomato I little squares. Mix in a bowl the tuna, the boiled corn, parsley, olive oil, tomato and onions. Dress with salt and pepper. Fill the tomato holes with the mixture and decorate the top with a parsley leave. Serve over lettuce leaves.

Nutritional facts: Energy 141 kcal, proteins 9.5 g, total fat 4.8 g, cholesterol 3.5 mg, carbohydrates 18.3 g, fiber 4.6 g and sodium 287 mg.

4.   Paella with vegetables

Ingredients:

- 2 cups of rice

- 1 eggplant cut in cubes

- 5 tomatoes cut and peeled

- 1 onion cut by the half

- 1 yellow pepper cut in strips

- 1 red pepper cut in strips

- 2 spoons of milled pepper

- salt

- 6 spoons of olive oil

- 1 garlic teeth

- 3 cups of chicken consommé

- black pepper

- 1 saffron stick

- 1 cup of mushrooms

- 1 cup of kidney beans

- 2 cups of cooked chickpeas

Procedure: Dissolve the saffron stick on 3 spoons of vegetable consommé. Put the eggplant in water with salt for 30 minutes and then stir. In a big pan warm the oil and Styr-fry the onion, garlic, pepper and eggplant for 5 minutes. Move from time to time. Pour the milled pepper and move again. Add the rice, the consommé, tomatoes and saffron, move again. Dress and let it boil. Once it is boiling reduce the fire and let it cook for another 15 minutes. Add the mushrooms, kidney beans and chickpeas. Keep boiling for another 10 minutes. Serve warm. To make the vegetable consommé put in a pot the carrots, celery and pepper. Cover them with water, add salt and let it boil covered for 20 minutes.

Nutritional facts: Energy 367 kcal, protein 11.1 g, total fat 9.6 g, cholesterol 0 mg, carbohydrates 61.6 g, fiber 8.9 g and sodium 364 mg.

5. Pear compote, lactose free milk and whole meal bread with cheese

Ingredients:

- 1 kg of pear
- 1 cinnamon stick
- little sugar if necessary
- 1 glass of lactose free milk
- 2 slices of whole meal bread
- 3 slices of cheese

Procedure:

Peel the pears, cut them in six pieces and take the seeds out. Cook it in bowling water for 15 minutes with the cinnamon stick inside. If you want add a little sugar and let it cool.

Serve one glass of lactose free milk with whole meal bread and three slices of cheese.

Nutritional facts: Energy 429 kcal, protein 17.3 g, total fat 3.7 g, cholesterol 8.1 mg, carbohydrates 85.5 g, fiber 8.6 g and sodium 563 mg.

6.   Tomato and potato crème soup (for 8 people)

Ingredients:

- 2 spoons of olive oil

- 1 big onion

- 4 mid-sized tomatoes

- 2 medium potatoes

- 2 spoons of chives

- 1 spoon of tomato sauce

- 1 liter of chicken consommé

- 1 spoon of grated lemon

- 1/2 spoon of thyme

- 1 laurel leave

- pepper

- thyme to decorate

Procedure: Peel the potatoes, onions and tomatoes next to the chives. Heat the oil in a pot and fry the onion until it is soft. Add the tomatoes, potatoes, chives, tomato sauce, grated lemon, thyme, laurel and chicken consommé. Let it boil without a cover for 20 minutes. Put it away the fire and take the laurel out and let it cool. Put the soup in the blender and mix until you get a creamy look. Put it again in the pot, dress with salt and pepper. Serve and decorate with thyme.

Nutritional facts: Energy 265 kcal, protein 9.4 g, total fat 7.2 g, cholesterol 27.6 mg, carbohydrates 48 g, fiber 7.8 g and sodium 153 mg.

7. Melon, tea with lactose free milk, toasted bread with low calories jam

Ingredients:

- 1 cup of melon cut on squares

- 1/2 cup of lactose free milk

- 1/2 cup of tea

- 2 toasted bread

- 3 slices of cheese

- 3 spoons of low calories jam

Procedure: A cup of melon cut on little squares, one big cup of lactose free milk with tea, two toasted bread with cheese and low calories jam.

Nutritional facts: Energy 242 kcal, proteins 14.8 g, total at 3.6 g, cholesterol 8.1 mg, carbohydrates 38.6 g, fiber 2.9 g and sodium 357.4 mg.

8.   Yogurt with apples and dried fruits

Ingredients:

- 1 apple
- 125 g of lactose free milk
- 5 almonds
- 5 raisins
- 5 nuts

Procedure: Peel the apple and cut it in little squares, mix with lactose free yogurt (125 g). Serve with 5 almonds, 5 raisins and 5 nuts.

Nutritional facts: Energy 264 kcal, proteins 9.5 g, total fat 10.2 g, cholesterol 16 mg, carbohydrates 29.1 g, fiber 3.3 g and sodium 101.2 mg.

9. Kiwi juice, lactose free yogurt and oats

Ingredients:

- 3 kiwis

- 1/2 cup of water

- 2 spoons of sugar

- 125 g of lactose free

- 2 spoons of oats

Procedure: Put 3 kiwis in the blender with half cup of water, and a little sugar if necessary. In another cup serve lactose free yogurt (125 g) with three spoons of oats.

Nutritional facts: Energy 297 kcal, proteins 13.4 g, total fat 1.7 g, cholesterol 2.7 mg, carbohydrates 58.9 g, fiber 7.5 g and sodium 376 mg.

10.   Plums, milk with coffee, bread with avocado

Ingredients:

- 2 plums

- 1 cup of lactose free milk

- 2 spoons of coffee

- 2 slices of white bread

- 1/2 avocado

Procedure: Two plums, a cup of coffee with lactose free milk and two slices of white bread with half avocado cut in slices. If you wish you can also smash the avocado with a fork and make a sauce of it, and then spread it on the bread.

Nutritional facts: Energy 288 kcal, proteins 16 g, total fat 3 g, cholesterol 5 mg, carbohydrates 52.1 g, fiber 5.6 g and sodium 502 mg.

11.   Strawberry with mint

Ingredients:

- 1 cup of lactose free milk

- 2 spoons of coffee

- 2 slices of whole meal bread

- 2 spoons of low carb jelly

- 1 cup of strawberry with mint leaves.

Procedure: Serve the milk with the coffee and pour the jelly over the bread. Cut the strawberries and put them in a pot, pour mint on top.

Nutritional facts: Energy 30 kcal, proteins 0 g, total fat 0g, cholesterol 70.3 mg, carbohydrates 7 g, fiber 2 g and sodium 1 mg.

12.   Mixed Salad (for six people)

Ingredients:

- 1 lettuce cut in strips

- 1/2 cup of carrots cut in julienne style

- 1 tomato cut in little squares

- 1/2 bundle of cut chives

Dressing:

- 1 cup of ricotta cheese

- 1 cup of natural yogurt (125 g)

- 1 bundle of chives

- Salt and pepper

Vinaigrette:

- 1/4 cup of olive oil

- 1/4 cup of balsamic vinegar

- Salt and pepper

Procedure: For dressing mix in the blender ricotta, yogurt, salt, pepper and chives. In a bowl mix all the other ingredients of the salad, add the vinaigrette and mix. Put the dressing on top and decorate with chives.

Nutritional facts: Energy 56 kcal, proteins 1.4 g, total fat 3.3 g, cholesterol 54 mg, carbohydrates 6.5 g, fiber 2.1 g and sodium 134 mg.

13. Filled meat balls (for 6 people)

Ingredients:

- 1/2 kg of ground beef

- 1/2 onion cut in little squares

- Salt and pepper

- 2 ½ cup of corn

- 2 ½ cup of peas

Procedure:

With few drops of olive oil sauté the onions in the pan, mix with the ground beef, salt and pepper. Form meat balls with this mixture. With the back part of a spoon flatten the center of each meat ball. In the space we just made add the corn, peas and few drops of olive oil. Put the filled meat balls in the oven on regular fire for ½ hour.

Nutritional facts: Energy 293 kcal, protein 25.4 g, total fat 6.5 g, cholesterol 56.7 mg, carbohydrates 33.1 g, fiber 4.9 g and sodium 277 mg.

14.   Traffic light of ice cream (for 6 people)

Ingredients:

- 4 bananas

- 8 ice cream sticks

- 4 balls of melon

- 4 balls of peach

- 4 balls of watermelon

Procedure:

Cut the bananas by half. Insert in each an ice cream stick. Decorate with the fruit balls cut by the half, put the watermelon on the top, peach in the middle and at the bottom the melon pretending to create a traffic light. Take it to the fridge for 1 hour.

Nutritional facts: Energy 102 kcal, proteins 1.2 g, total fat 0.4 g, cholesterol 0 mg, carbohydrates 17.8 gr and sodium 3 mg.

15.   Little forms of corn flour (for 6 people)

Ingredients:

- 6 cups of water

- 1/2 cup of salt

- 2 cups of corn flour

- 2 spoons of olive oil

Sauce:

- 1 cup of lactose free milk

- 1 spoon of oil

- 1 spoon of flour

- 1/2 cup of tomato sauce

Procedure: Put the water with salt in a pot until it boils. Reduce the fire and add the corn flour as rain. Mix continuously with a wood spoon for a minute. Add the olive oil and mix. Pour the mixture in an oven platter that has been already bath in oil. Smooth the surface with a wet a spatula and let it cool. Cut with a cookie breaker or with a knife in squares of 2x2 centimeters. Prepare the white sauce by warming the spoon of oil and adding the flour; let it cook for five minutes. Add to the sauce the boiling cup of milk and move constantly so it won't stick. Then mix it with the tomato sauce. Cook the corn flour forms we got before with the sauce on top in the oven, make sure you cover completely the oven platter in order not to dry the food.

Nutritional facts: energy 241 kcal, protein 7.9 g, total fat 5.8 g, cholesterol 6.5 mg, carbohydrates 40.7 g, fiber 5.9 g and sodium 342 mg.

16.   Bean and tomato salad (for 6 people)

Ingredients:

- 3 mid-size tomatoes

- 2 cups of green beans

- salt

- 2 spoons of olive oil

Procedure: Peel the tomatoes and cut in little squares. Peel the green beans and cut in julienne style, make them boil in little water and make sure not to cover the pot so the beans will keep its color. Mix and dress with oil and salt.

Nutritional facts: Energy 53 kcal, protein 0.3 g, total fat 3.3 g, cholesterol 0 mg, carbohydrates 4.6 g, fiber 0.6 g and sodium 339 mg.

17.   Mix of fruits and lactose free yogurt (4 people)

Ingredients:

- 1 cup of melon
- 1 cup of fruit mix (peach, apple and watermelon)
- 15 cherries
- 1 yogurt

Procedure: Mix in a bowl the melon, the fruit-mix that has been cut in slices, the cherries and 1 yogurt (125 g). Serve in little dessert cups.

Nutritional facts: energy 99 kcal, protein 4.1 g, total fat 0.9 g, cholesterol 0.1 mg, carbohydrates 20.6 g, fiber 3.8 g and sodium 41.1 mg.

18.   Cauliflower cream (for 6 people)

Ingredients:

- 750 g of cauliflower

- 1 cup of cut onion in little squares

- 200 g of almonds

- 800 ml of chicken consommé

- 3 spoons of olive oil

- salt and pepper

- 2 chives

Procedure: Peel the almonds and toast them in the oven for five minutes. Warm the oil in a pot, add the cut onion and brown it, add the cauliflower and the chicken consommé. Boil everything together and cover it, for 25 minutes. Mix in the blender, the soup with the almonds, to get a cream and put it back to the pot. Add salt and pepper.

Nutritional facts: Energy 66 kcal, protein 2.77 g, total fat 3.7 g, cholesterol 18.7 mg, carbohydrates 7 g, fiber 2.6 g and sodium 200 mg.

19.   Cobb Salad (for 6 people)

Ingredients:

- 1 lettuce cut in strips

- 1 cup of tomatoes in cubes

- 1 cup of avocado cut in cubes

- 1 cup of cooked grains of corn

- 3 cooked eggs (separate yolk from white)

- 2 cooked chicken filet cut in cubes or turkey chest or a can of tuna.

- 1/4 cup of wine vinaigrette

- 1/4 cup of natural yogurt

- 1/4 cup of milk

- Salt

Procedure: Mix in the blender vinaigrette, milk, natural yogurt and salt. Put this dressing on all the ingredients by separate and put in a round platter on layers, first the lettuce, then the tomatoes, avocado, corn and chicken. Put the eggs on top of the tower. To decorate add some dressing on the top. You can also build the towers on individual dishes if necessary.

Nutritional facts: Energy 189 kcal, protein 18.2 g, total fat 9.1 g, cholesterol 70.3 mg, carbohydrates 10.4 g, fiber 4.8 g and sodium 332 mg.

20. Faustus salad (for ten people)

Ingredients:

- 2 cups of Peeled tomatoes cut in small cubes
- 2 cups of avocado in small cubes
- 2 cups of corn
- 1/4 cup of onion rings
- 2 spoons of fine cut of parsley
- 2 spoons of fine cut of coriander
- 1 spoon of salt
- 2 spoons of vinaigrette
- 1 spoon of lemon juice

Dressing:

- 3 spoons of vinaigrette
- 9 spoons of olive oil
- 1 spoon of fine cut of parsley
- 1 spoon of mustard

Procedure: Peel the tomatoes and cut them, add 1 spoon of salt, 2 spoons of vinaigrette and put everything on a strainer to dry. Cook the corn and add one spoon of salt. Peel and cut the avocado. In a glass bowl, put 1 cut tomato, over all a layer of avocado and onion, add salts. Cover all with the corn. Then repeat the procedure and pour the dressing over it, decorate with the cut parsley.

Nutritional facts: Energy 134 kcal, proteins 2.9 g, total fat 8.6 g, cholesterol 15 mg, carbohydrates 15.3 g, fiber 7.3 g and sodium 216 mg.

21. Tuna omelet (for two people)

Ingredients:

- 1 can of tuna on water

- 2 eggs

- salt and oil

Procedure: Separate the yolk from the white of the eggs, shake the white for two minutes. Then add the yolk and salt. Separate the tuna form the water, and then mix the tuna with the eggs. Warm the pan with olive oil, when it is warm pour the mixture, distribute it uniformly. Cook the omelet for 5 minutes, turn it around by helping yourself with a pot top and let the other side cook for another five minutes.

Nutritional facts: Energy 203 kcal, proteins 24.2 g, total fat 9.9 g, cholesterol 233.3 mg, carbohydrates 2 g, fiber 0 g and sodium 506 mg.

22.   Ceviche of salmon, avocado and lettuce (for six people)

Ingredients:

- 3 cups of salmon cut in cubes
- 1 onion cut on julienne style
- olive oil
- dried dill
- chives
- red or green chili
- 1/4 of spoon of ginger powder
- 1/4 of cup of lemon juice
- 1 cucumber
- sesame seeds

Avocado cream:

- 2 spoons of fine cuts of coriander
- 2 avocados
- 1/2 natural yogurt
- lettuce

Procedure: Boil water in one pot, reduce the fire to the minimum and cook the salmon cut in cubes for ten minutes. Take all the water out. Peel and cut the onion on julienne style. Cut the chili, the sesame seed and the chives. In a bowl, mix the onion with the olive oil, lemon juice, dried dill, ginger, chives and cooked salmon. For the avocado cream, peel and cut the avocado in cubes and mix with the coriander and yogurt. Cut the cucumber on layers. In a metal bowl put half of the salmon mixture, then add a layer of cucumber and another layer of salmon. Finish with a layer of avocado cream. Decorate with sesame seeds and chives. Join it with lettuce salad.

Nutritional facts: Energy 249 kcal, proteins 23.4 g, total fat 13.4 g, cholesterol 52.8 mg, carbohydrates 9.9 g, fiber 4.5 g and sodium 291 mg.

23.   Peppers cream (for 6 people)

Ingredients:

- 1 ½ kg of red pepper

- 1 liter of chicken consommé

- 2 little spoons of curry

- 1 natural yogurt low in calories and without sugar

- salt and pepper

- grated cheese to decorate

Procedure: Wash and peel the pepper. Cook the chicken consommé with the curry for 30 minutes. Mix everything in the blender. Strain and put all back in the blender. Add the yogurt until it has a creamy look. Add to the mixture salt and pepper and then serve. Decorate with grated cheese.

Nutritional facts: Energy 57 kcal, protein 3.6 g, total fat 1.1 gr, cholesterol 19 mg, carbohydrates 9.6 gr, fiber 2 g and sodium 317 mg.

24.   Lettuce salad, beef with broad beans warm salad

Ingredients:

- 4 beef filets low in fat (ball back or steak)
- salt and oregano
- 4 cups of lettuce
- parsley
- 4 cups of broad beans
- 1 onion

Procedure: Cook the beef filets with a minimum of olive oil and condiments. Cook the broad beans and cut the onions in little squares and stir-fry it. Mix the onions and serve the beef filets with the warm broad beans with the lettuce salad and parsley to decorate.

Nutritional facts: Energy 379 kcal, protein 30.3 gr, total fat 10.3 g, cholesterol 0.2 mg, carbohydrates 53.1 g, fiber 6.3 g and sodium 452.4 mg.

25.   Creole salad (for 8 people)

Ingredients:

- 1 lettuce

- 200 g of spinach (only leaves)

- 2 spoons of coriander in fine cuts

- 3/4 cup of onion rings

- 4 cooked eggs

- 2 avocado

- 1 ½ cups of tomato

Dressing:

- 3 spoons of vinaigrette

- 9 spoons of oil

- 1 spoon of cut parsley

- 1/2 spoons of dried tarragon

- 1 spoon of mustard

Procedure: Wash the lettuce and spinach, cut with hand. In a salad bowl put the mixture of lettuce, spinach and coriander. Cut the avocado in strips and put it as a fan in the middle of the salad bowl. Cut the eggs in quarters and put them in a row next to the avocado. Peel the tomatoes, take the seeds out and cut in small squares. Put the tomato around the eggs. Pour the dressing on top and add while serving.

Nutritional facts: Energy 115 kcal, protein 4g, total fat 9.3 g, cholesterol 70.7 mg, carbohydrates 5.9 g, fiber 4.6 g and sodium 113 mg.

26.   Chicken with coriander and rice with pepper (for 4 people)

Ingredients:

- 1/2 kilo of chicken filet
- 1 spoon of grains of black pepper
- 2 spoons of ginger powder
- 1 bundle of cut coriander
- 1/2 onion cut in squares
- scrape one lemon
- 400 ml of coconut milk
- 4 leaves of lemon
- some leaves of basil

Procedure: Smash the ginger with the pepper grains. Add the fresh condiments, coriander, scrape of lemon and onion and smash them until you get a paste. Fry the paste in a pan with chicken consommé, add coconut milk and lemon leaves, and cook with slowly fire for ten minutes. In another pot cook the chicken in water with salt. Let it cool and cut the chicken in cubes of 3 cm, distribute them in a font and serve the sauce over it.

The coconut milk can be bought or cooked at home. For this you have to boil 400 ml of lactose free milk and a coconut package. Turn off the fire. Cover the pot and let it rest for 20 minutes and then strain.

Nutritional facts: Energy 438 kcal, protein 22.2 g, total fat 11.2 g, cholesterol 36.2 mg, carbohydrates 58.1 g, fiber 3.6 g and sodium 206 mg.

For rice with pepper: 2 cups of white rice, 1 garlic teeth, 1 cup of red pepper and salt.

Mix the pepper in the blender. In a pot, mix the garlic and the rice on low fire; add the pepper sauce and immediately 4 cups of boiling water and salt. Cook with minimum fire.

Nutritional facts: Energy 165 kcal, proteins 2.8 g, total fat 0.8 g, cholesterol 0 mg, carbohydrates 34 g, fiber 0.8 g and sodium 69.5 mg.

27.   Funny salad (for 6 people)

Ingredients:

- 1 ½ cup of cauliflower

- 1/2 cup of black olives

- 1 ½ spoons of cut pepper

- 1/4 of onion cut in little squares

- 1/2 spoon of oregano

- 2 spoons of vinaigrette

- 1/2 cup of olive oil

- 1 drop of spicy chili

- 2 spoons of parmesan grated cheese

- 5 cups of lettuce on a fine cut

Procedure: Put all the ingredients together in a salad pot, besides the lettuce, and mix. Before serving add the lettuce and mix again.

Nutritional facts: Energy 74 kcal, proteins 1.3 g, total fat 6.9 g, cholesterol 0 mg, carbohydrates 3.1 g, fiber 1.4 g and sodium 246 mg.

28.   Crown of artichoke with spring rice (for 6 people)

Ingredients:

- 6 slices of cooked turkey chest
- 1 onion cut in little squares
- 1 spoon of olive oil
- 1 cup of cooked artichoke (5 artichokes)
- 4 eggs
- 1 cup of lactose free milk powder
- 3/4 cups of parmesan grated cheese
- salt and pepper
- 1/4 spoon of nutmeg

Procedure: Pre-warm the oven on 200°C. Put oil in the crown mold. Cover the interior with the turkey. Let some parts of the turkey to hang outside to cover the mixture once is full. In another pan, fry the onions with oil till it is soft and take it away from the fire.

In the blender mix the artichoke. Add the eggs one by one and then the milk powder, cheese and onion. Condiment with salt and mix again. Pour the mixture in the mold and cover with the turkey sides and the rest on top. Put the mold on water bath and bake it for 30 minutes or till a knife comes out after sticking it inside. Serve cold with yogurt sauce and parsley, or warm with white sauce.

Spring rice for 8 people

Ingredients:

- 2 cups of rice
- 1/2 cups of corn
- 1/2 cups of peas
- 1 carrot
- 1 spoon of salt

Procedure: Stir-fry the rice, move constantly, this way no oil is necessary. When the grain is a little brown, add corn, peas and carrots in squares, salt and 4 cups of boiling water. Cook with slowly fire for 20 minutes.

Nutritional facts (including the rice): Energy 342 kcal, proteins 15.9 g, total fat 5.6 g, cholesterol 81.9 mg, carbohydrates 57.9 g, fiber 9.1 g and sodium 344 mg.

29.   Salad of kidney beans, tomato, lettuce and avocado (for 4 people)

Ingredients:

-   2 cups of lettuce

-   1 avocado

-   2 tomatoes

-   2 cups of green cooked kidney beans

Procedure: Peel the tomatoes and cut them in little squares, take out the points of the kidney beans and cut in julienne style, cook them for 10 minutes in boiling water without covering and then let them cool. Cut the lettuce and avocado in cubes, mix all together and dress as you like the most.

Nutritional facts: Energy 78.1 kcal, proteins 2.3 g, total fat 4.5 g, cholesterol 0 mg, carbohydrates 8.8 g, fiber 4.9 g and sodium 162 mg.

30.   Noodles with Bolognese sauce

Bolognese sauce: (for 6-8 people)

Ingredients:

- 1 onion

- 1 carrot

- 250 g of ground beef

- 2 cups of natural tomato sauce

- 2 spoons of dried oregano

- 1/4 of boiling water

- salt and pepper

Procedure:

Cut the onion in squares and fry in a pan with a spoon of olive oil. When onion is soft add the carrots and stir-fry till its soft, too. Add the beef and cook moving from time to time. Add the salt, pepper and oregano. Add the tomato sauce, let it boil and add boiling water so we get a juicy sauce. Boil noodles and join them with the sauce.

Nutritional facts: Energy 404 kcal, proteins 14.3 g, total fat 5.8 g, cholesterol 52.9 mg, carbohydrates 72.9 g, fiber 6.1 g and sodium 236 mg.

31. Tomato salad with cucumber and cabbage with coriander (for 4 people)

Ingredients:

- 2 tomatoes

- 1 cucumber

- 2 cups of cabbage

- coriander

- lemon

- salt and oil

Procedure: Wash and peel the cucumber, make long cuts by the half, take out the seeds with a spoon and then cut in slices. Peel the tomato, cut in squares and mix with the cucumber. Cut the cabbage leaves in julienne style and mix with the coriander. Use your favorite dressing.

Nutritional facts: Energy 61 kcal, protein 1.8 g, total fat 2.8 g, cholesterol 0 mg, carbohydrates 9.1 g, fiber 3 g and sodium 213 mg.

32.   Beef stew (for 4 people)

Ingredients:

- 2 spoons of olive oil

- 6 pieces of beef (roast)

- 6 pieces of corn

- 6 pieces of squash

- 6 little potatoes

- 1 cup of cut onion in squares

- 1 carrot cut in squares

- 1/2 red pepper cut in julienne style

- 3 spoons of rice

- 1 cup of peas

- enough water to cover the beef pieces

- 8 spoons of coriander as powder

- salt and pepper

Procedure: Warm the oil and stir-fry the onion, carrot and red pepper. When the vegetables are soft, brown the beef pieces on it. Add water till it covers the beef pieces (750 ml), dress with salt and pepper. Cover the top, turn down the fire and cook for 40 minutes, until the beef is cook and soft. Add the corn, potatoes and cooks for 20 more minutes. 5 minutes before finishing add the squash pieces, peas and rice. Add boiling water if necessary and keep the top covered. Verify the level of salt. Sprinkle the cut coriander while serving.

Nutritional facts: Energy 375 kcal, proteins 28.4 g, total fat 6.2 g, cholesterol 68.1 mg, carbohydrates 45.5 g, fiber 5 g and sodium 285 mg.

33.   Exotic salad (for 4 people)

Ingredients:

- 200 g of mix lettuce

- 200 g of spinach leaves

- 1 tangerine

- 50 g of toasted almonds cut in slices

- 1 avocado in strips

Dressing:

- 3 spoons of apple vinegar

- 2 spoons of honey

- 1/2 cups of evaporated milk

- 1/4 cup of olive oil

- salt and pepper

Procedure: Put the spinach and lettuce in a salad bowl, mix and put the avocado on top, tangerine and almonds. Prepare the dressing mixing all the ingredients in the blender. Pour over the salad while serving.

Nutritional facts: Energy 94 kcal, protein 2 g, total fat 6.4 g, cholesterol 2.3 mg, carbohydrates 8.9 g, fiber 2.7 g and sodium 225 mg.

34.   Mongolian beef with brown rice (for 4 people)

Ingredients:

- 250 g of steak
- 1 onion
- 1 cup of cut chives
- 1 red pepper and 1 green pepper
- 1 green chili
- 3/4 cups of water
- salt and dressing, pepper

Procedure: Cut the onions in julienne style with the green part of the chives and sliced the white part. Also cut the pepper in julienne style and sliced the chili. Add all the ingredients and sauté in a deep pan. Once the vegetables are soft add the water and cover to get juice. Separately cut the beef in triangles and grill. Once the beef is ready dress with salt, pepper and additional dressing as you want. Join both mixtures and add boiling water if necessary.

Brown rice (for 6 people)

Ingredients:

- 2 cups of brown rice

- 2 eggs

- chives

- 2 cups of chicken in cubes

- salt

- 1/2 onion

Procedure: Cut the onion in squares and fry. Before it goes brown add the rice and sauté, then add 4 cups of boiling water, salt and cook with low fire. Shake the eggs with a fork, cook them as an omelet, and do not fry. When it is cold cut it in strips. Grill the chicken and cut. Cut the chives in slices. When rice is done join everything in a wok and mix again.

Nutritional facts (including rice and beef): Energy 413 kcal, protein 19.5 g, total fat 10.5 g, cholesterol 75.5 mg, carbohydrates 58.6 g, fiber 2.8 g and sodium 330 mg.

35.   Crunchy chicken with potato purée (for 4 people)

Ingredients:

- 6 pieces of chicken

- 40 g of grated bread

- 40 g of smashed almonds

- 4 spoons of fine herbs

- 1/2 liter of chicken consommé

- parsley and thyme

- salt and pepper

Procedure: Clean the chicken by taking the fat away, also the skin must go out, add salt and pepper. Put the chicken in a grill over a baking dish inside the oven. Mix the grated bread, almonds and fine herbs and cover the chicken. Put in the bottom of the oven the chicken consommé with the fine herbs to give aroma. Cook in the pre-warmed oven under moderate fire for 40 minutes.

Potato purée (for 4 people)

Ingredients:

- 6 potatoes from the same size

- salt

- 4 spoons of olive oil

- 300 ml of lactose free milk

Procedure: Peel the potatoes and cook in water with salt for 20 minutes, since water start to boil. Then smash the potatoes with the help of a press while they are warm. Add the olive oil and shake with an electric mixer till potatoes are soft. Try the salt level and add more if necessary. Warm the mixture in a pot and keep mixing, add slowly the warm milk. Serve when the mixture is hot. If you need to warm it again you must do it in a pot, never in the microwave, move with a wood spoon and add warm milk if necessary.

Nutritional facts (including the chicken and potatoes): Energy 348 kcal, proteins 32.8 gr, total fat 8.3 g, cholesterol 88.7 mg, carbohydrates 36 g, fiber 3.5 g and sodium 378 mg.

36. Cold rolls of filled potato purée (for 6 people)

Ingredients:

- 6 regular potatoes
- 1 cup of lactose free milk
- 1 cup of tuna
- 1 cup of peas
- 100 g of black olives
- 2 tomatoes cut in little squares
- 1 boiled egg
- salt
- pepper cut in julienne style
- 1 cup of boiled corn
- lettuce salad and tomato to join

Procedure: Prepare the purée with the potatoes, milk and salt. Make a layer of 1 cm with the purée over a thin wet fabric on a flat fount, as a rectangle. Distribute over it, on layers, the peas and tuna, pepper cut in julienne style, corn and olives. Roll it by helping you with the wet fabric and take it out slowly. Cut the borders and translate it again to the fount. Decorate with sliced eggs, olives and pepper.

Keep it in the fridge and serve it with lettuce and tomato salad.

Nutritional facts: Energy 294 kcal, protein 13.1 g, total fat 8.3 g, cholesterol 39.4 mg, carbohydrates 44.2 g, fiber 5.8 g and sodium 298 mg.

37.   Conger soup (for 8 people)

Ingredients:

- 2 onions

- 1 big cup of tomatoes

- 1 cup of lactose free milk

- salt, pepper and laurel

- 1 full conger including the head

- 1 potato per person

Procedure: Buy the fish clean and without skin with the head aside. Fry the onion with olive oil. Condiment the fish and put it on a pot where it can be separate from the consommé. Put on layers the onion, tomatoes and fish and repeat again the procedure. Add the head of the fish to give taste. Add the peeled potatoes and condiment with salt and pepper. Cook it on slowly fire, without the cover. Take out the fish head and while serving add the milk.

Nutritional facts: Energy 343 kcal, proteins 40.8 g, total fat 7.6 g, cholesterol 78.5 mg, carbohydrates 26.7 g, fiber 2.6 g and sodium 302 mg.

38.   Waldorf salad (for 6 people)

Ingredients:

- 4 cups of celery

- 3 green apples

- 6 nuts

- 4 spoons of natural lactose free yogurt

- juice of half lemon

- Salt and pepper

Procedure: Clean the celery and cut in thin slices. Cut the apples in dice shape and pour lemon juice over them. Cut the nuts and mix everything. Add salt and pepper to the yogurt and join all together.

Nutritional facts: Energy 99 kcal, protein 2.2 g, total fat 4.2 g, cholesterol 0.2 mg, carbohydrates 15.4 g, fiber 3,1 g and sodium 207 mg.

39.   Rice with seafood mussels

Ingredients:

- 4 dozens of mussels

- 4 cups of cooked white rice

- 2 spoons of cut onion in squares

- 2 yellow chilies (optional)

- 4 spoons of coriander purée

- 2 cups of mussel's consommé

- 1/2 cup of peas

- 1/2 cup of broad beans

- 1/2 cup of boiled corn

- parsley

- coriander

- olive oil

- salt and pepper

Procedure: Wash the mussels really good. Put them in a pot with parsley leaves and half cup of water. Cook with the top covered for 5 minutes till the shells are open. Strain and reserve the consommé. Take out the shells and keep the seafood clean. Wash the chilies and cut, take out the seeds and cut in julienne style. Prepare a purée with coriander, leaves of coriander and a little water in a blender. Boil the corn, broad beans and peas. Warm the oil in a wok, add the onions, yellow chilies and coriander purée, stir-fry and add the rice, mix till everything is together. Add the mussel consommé, cooked vegetables and seafood. Add salt and pepper to give flavor. Cook all together with low fire and decorate with coriander leaves while serving.

Nutritional facts: Energy 338 kcal, proteins 16.9 g, total fat 6.3 g, cholesterol 42.1 mg, carbohydrates 49.2 g, fiber 2.1 g and sodium 256 mg.

40.   Filled avocado with tuna and lettuce salad (for 4 people)

Ingredients:

- 4 avocados

- 1 can of tuna in water

- 2 cups of lettuce

- salt, oil and lemon

Procedure: Cut the avocado by the half, on the long side, peel and fill with tuna, serve over cut lettuce in julienne style.

Nutritional facts: Energy 143 kcal, proteins 10.7 g, total fat 1.5 g, cholesterol 5.4 mg, carbohydrates 5.6 g, fiber 6.3 g and sodium 215 mg.

41.   Lettuce with herbs sauce and noodles with tomato and basil

Ingredients:

- 1 lettuce
- 1 bundle of chives
- 1 spoon of parsley
- 1 spoon of basil
- 1 spoon of oregano
- 1 spoon of olive oil
- salt and pepper

Procedure: Cut the fine herbs and mix with the olive oil. Dress the lettuce cut in julienne style.

Nutritional facts: Energy 35 kcal, proteins 0.5 g, total fat 1.6 g, cholesterol 0 mg, carbohydrates 1.1 g, fiber 0.6 g and sodium 213 mg.

Noodles (for 4 people)

Ingredients:

- 300 g of noodles

Sauce:

- 1 cup of tomato sauce

- 1/2 kg of tomato cut in squares

- 1 onion

- 2 spoons of olive oil

- 10 basil leaves

- 50 g of black olives

- salt and pepper in grain

Procedure: Cook the noodles; wash them in cold water so it won't stick and reserve aside. For the dressing, cut the onion in small squares, add the oil and the tomato sauce and cook for 5 minutes. Turn off the fire and add the fresh cut tomatoes, basil leaves and olives. Add salt pepper to give flavor and add the noodles on the pan and mix with the sauce. Move the pan so the noodles won't crush and serve with some just smashed pepper on top.

Nutritional facts: Energy 404 kcal, proteins 12.2 g, total fat 9.8 g, cholesterol 0 mg, carbohydrates 68.2 g, fiber 8.1 g and sodium 332 mg.

42.   Avocado mousse (for 8 people)

Ingredients:

- 4 avocados

- 1 lemon

- 2 white eggs

- 4 spoons of natural yogurt

- 5 little spoons of powder jelly

- 1 tomato to decorate

- 1 kg of green kidney beans

- salt and pepper

Procedure: Peel the avocado and smash them, add the lemon juice and the yogurt. Shake the white eggs till snow point and reserve aside. Incorporate the jelly powder and mix with the avocado cream, then mix with the eggs. Bath the mold with oil and cover it with transparent paper, then put a layer of tomatoes and cover with the avocado purée. Cover with film and put it in the fridge for 6 hours. Serve and join it with boiled kidney beans on top.

Nutritional facts: energy 262 kcal, protein 10.3 g, total fat 18.9 g, cholesterol 1.8 mg, carbohydrates 16.8 g, fiber 10.4 g and sodium 382 mg.

43.　　Pancakes filled with spinach (10 und.)

Pancakes:

- 2 cups of milk

- 2 eggs

- 1 ½ cups of flour

Fill:

- 1 bundle of spinach

- 2 spoons of olive oil

- 3 spoons of flour

- 1/2 liter of lactose free milk

- salt, pepper and nutmeg

Procedure: Prepare the pancakes, join and shake the ingredients, put the mixture in thin layer on a pan and fry. Pan must be warm before it. Wash the spinach leaves, and with that same water take it to the microwave and cook it for 1 minute. Now put it immediately on cold water to keep a nice color. Cut them in thin strips or mix in a blender and reserve aside. Prepare the white sauce, put the olive oil in a pot and mix with flour. Cut the fire, add a little milk and solve it by using a wood spoon. Turn on the fire and let it boil while moving constantly to avoid the formation of lumps. Integrate the sauce and the spinach and fill the pancakes. Reserve a little of white sauce without spinach to pour on the pancakes. You can roll the pancake or little packages with them, tied them with chives leaves.

Nutritional facts (for 2 units): Energy 234 kcal, proteins 11.8 g, total fat 6.5 g, cholesterol 63.1 mg, carbohydrates 32.5 g, fiber 3.2 g and sodium 369 mg.

44.   Salad with cabbage, carrots and peanuts (for 5 people)

Ingredients:

- 3 cups of white cabbage

- 3 cups of purple cabbage

- 3 carrots

- 1/2 cup of peanuts

- salt, oil and lemon

Procedure: Cut the cabbage in julienne style and wash the carrots; mix with peanuts and dress.

Nutritional facts: Energy 68 kcal, protein 1.9 g, total fat 4.1 g, cholesterol 0 mg, carbohydrates 6 g, fiber 2.3 g and sodium 225.8 mg.

45. Chicken with honey and rice with squash (for 6 people)

Ingredients:

- 6 chicken pieces

- 6 spoons of palm honey

- 1 little spoon of salt

- 1 little spoon of mustard

- 1 little spoon of curry powder

Procedure: Put all the ingredients, besides the chicken, in a pot. Warm and mix. Put the chicken pieces, washed and without skin or fat and cover, on another pot and cover it with the sauce. Bake it at 180°C or mid temperature for 1 hour, until the chicken is soft and brown.

For the rice:

Ingredients:

- 1 cup of white rice

- 1 onion cut in little squares

- 3 spoons of olive oil

- 1/2 chicken chest

- 2 spoons of squash cooked and smashed

- 2 spoons of boiled corn

- 2 spoons of boiled peas

- fresh oregano

- salt and pepper

Procedure: Warm the olive oil in a pot, add the onions and Styr-fry and while it is still colorful add the rice and the squash purée. Rice must be white because it has the perfect consistency for this recipe. Add the chicken consommé, for this cook the chicken chest without skin in little water. Let it cool and take the fat out, add salt and pepper. Cook on low fire for 15 minutes. Take it out of the fire and separate the grains with a fork. Add the boiled corn and peas to the rice and mix. Serve and sprinkle oregano meanwhile.

Nutritional facts (considering chicken and rice): Energy 325 kcal, proteins 20.5 g, total fat 7.8 g, cholesterol 77.6 mg, carbohydrates 40.7 g, fiber 1.3 g and sodium 359 mg.

46.   Filled artichoke contour with kidney beans salad (for 4 people)

Ingredients:

- 4 artichokes

- 1/2 liter of natural yogurt

- coriander

- 4 cups of kidney beans

- salt, olive oil and lemon

Procedure: Cook the artichokes in boiling water for 30-40 minutes, separate the bottom from the leaves, take out the pulp from the bottom with a spoon and mix it with the yogurt and coriander. Dress the kidney beans with salt, olive oil and lemon; then put them on bottom of the artichokes and fill with everything else, with the sauce.

Nutritional facts: Energy 69 kcal, protein 5.1 g, total fat 3.3 g, cholesterol 0.3 mg, carbohydrates 14.8 g, fiber 10 g and sodium 239 mg.

47.   Grilled beef with herbs (for 8 people)

Ingredients:

- 1 kg of beef (steak)
- 2 spoons of fresh rosemary
- 2 spoons of fresh thyme
- 2 leaves of laurel
- 1/2 purple onion
- 1 spoon of orange zest
- 1 spoon of sea salt
- 1 spoon of milled black pepper
- 1/2 spoon of milled nutmeg
- 1 clove
- 2 spoons of olive oil
- 8 potatoes
- chives

Procedure: First we have to create a crust that covers the beef. For this mix all the ingredients in the blender until we reach a creamy look, then pour the mixture on the beef and let it rest for 6 hours. Pre-warm the oven. Bake the beef for 30 minutes. Take out of the oven and let it cool covered for

10 minutes, cut it in gross slices and add the juices from baking. Serve with boiled potatoes and chives.

Nutritional facts: Energy 320 kcal, proteins 32.9 g, total fat 5.9, cholesterol 10.2 mg, carbohydrates 32.7 g, fiber 2.2 g and sodium 398 mg.

48. Beetroot and carrot salad with turkey rolls with vegetables (for 6 people)

For Beetroot salad:

Ingredients:

- 3 beetroot

- 3 carrots

- salt, olive oil and lemon

Procedure: Peel the carrots and beetroot, grate, mix and dress as you like.

Nutritional facts: Energy 36 kcal, proteins 1.3 g, total fat 0.8 g, cholesterol 0 mg, carbohydrates 5.8 g, fiber 2.8 g and sodium 342.5 mg.

For the turkey rolls with vegetables:

Ingredients:

- 3/4 kg of spiral noodles

- 200 g of chest of turkey

- 1 carrot

- 1 green pepper

- 1 cup of boiled corn

- 1 cup of peas

- 1 onion cut in rings

- oregano

- salt and olive oil

Procedure: cut the turkey in cubes and sauté with a little oil, dress with salt and oregano. Add the pepper that has been previously cut in little squares, the boiled corn and peas, grate the carrots and add the onion rings. Cook for 3 minutes and fill he spirals with this mixture.

Nutritional facts: Energy 349 kcal, protein 19.2 g, total fat 2.7 g, cholesterol 38 mg, carbohydrates 59.2 g, fiber 6.3 g and sodium 251.2 mg.

49.　Gazpacho (for 6-8 people)

Ingredients:

- 3/4 kg of red tomatoes
- 1/2 onion
- 1 small green pepper
- 1 slide of whole meal bread
- 1 garlic teeth
- 4 spoons of olive oil
- 1/2 spoons of red wine vinegar
- 1 cup of cold water
- salt and pepper
- lemon juice

To serve:

- 1 tomato
- 1 cucumber
- 1 pepper
- 8 slices of bread toasted in the oven

Procedure: Peel the tomatoes, cut them by the half and take the seeds out. Peel the onion and cut in squares. Take out the seeds and veins from the green pepper. Cut the garlic by the half and separate the green center if there is one. Put everything together in the blender, besides the salt and lemon. Mix. Put the mixture in a bowl and add salt, pepper and lemon. Let it cool. If it is too dense add a little cold water. To serve prepare the tomato, cucumber and pepper: peeled, take out the seeds and cut in squares. Now add to every dish with the previous mixture.

Nutritional facts: Energy 156 kcal, proteins 3 g, total fat 6.8 g, cholesterol 0 mg, carbohydrates 19.4 g, fiber 2.3 g and sodium 303.7 mg.

50. Chicken with artichoke and brown rice (for 6 people)

Ingredients:

- 6 chicken pieces
- 8 hearts of artichoke with the fresh leaves inside
- 3 spoons of olive oil
- 1 cup of onion cut in squares
- 2 spoons of tomato sauce
- 1/4 cup of red wine vinegar
- 1 little spoon of sugar
- 1/2 cup of water
- 2 laurel leaves
- 2 spoons of parsley in fine cut
- salt and pepper
- lemon juice

Procedure: Warm the oil in a pot. Add salt and pepper to the chicken pieces and sauté until it is brown from every side, for 10 minutes. Take out and reserve. In another pot sauté the onions until they are brown. Add the tomato sauce and solve with the vinegar, move until it evaporates.

Add the sugar, ½ cup of water and laurel leaves. Add the chicken pieces to the pot and place them over the vegetables. Cover and let it cook over low fire for 30 minutes. Add the artichoke hearts and move slowly. Serve everything in a fount and pour parsley over all.

For the brown rice (for 6 people):

Ingredients:

-   2 cups of brown rice

-   2 ½ cups of water

-   salt

-   1 spoon of olive oil

Procedure: Wash the rice and strain it. In a pot warm the oil, and then add the water and salt. Cover the pot and let it boil. Add the rice and cover, once its boiling let it cook for 15 minutes. Separate the grains with a fork before serving.

Nutritional facts (chicken with rice): Energy 435 kcal, proteins 26 g, total fat 13.3 g, cholesterol 59.3 mg, carbohydrates 54.9 g, fiber 14.8 g and sodium 319 mg.

51.   Mexican fish (for 4 people)

Ingredients:

- 2 big tomatoes

- 1 onion

- 1 spoon of tomato sauce

- 1 spoon of cumin

- 1/2 spoon of coriander

- chili if you like

- 1/4 spoons of milled pepper

- 1 spoon of lemon juice

- 2 spoons of olive oil

- 4 fish filet

- 1/2 cup of grated cheese

Procedure: Cut the onion and the coriander. Peel the tomatoes, take out the seed and cut in little squares. Warm the oven on mid-term fire. Pour olive oil over the baking dish. Mix in a bowl the tomatoes, onion, tomato sauce, cumin, coriander and chili. In another bowl join together the pepper, lemon juice and olive oil. Put the fish filets on the baking dish. Pour the lemon sauce over each filet and cover with the tomato mixture. Pour the grated cheese on top and let it bake for 15 minutes.

Potato purée with basil

Ingredients:

- 1 bundle of basil
- ½ cup of olive oil
- 1 little spoon of mustard
- 1/2 kg o potatoes
- 1/4 of purple onion cut in squares
- 2 tomatoes on strips to decorate
- salt and pepper

Procedure: Cook the potatoes and make a purée with them. In boiling water put the basil leaves and take them out right away, let them cool with cold water. In a blender mix the basil leaves, olive oil, mustard, onion salt and pepper. Add the mixture to the purée and use an electric mixer to finish the purée.

Nutritional facts (fish and purée): Energy 424 kcal, protein 36.6 g, total fat 14 g, cholesterol 136 mg, carbohydrates 40.9 g, fiber 5.8 and sodium 385 mg.

52.   Chicken with orange and green rice (for 6 people)

Ingredients:

- 1 full chicken

- 6 laurel leaves

- 6 oranges

- 3 spoons of olive oil

- salt and pepper

Procedure: Condiment the chicken with salt and pepper. Put it in a baking dish and cover it with the laurel leaves. Bath the chicken with the orange juice and the oil. Bake it in a warm oven for 45 minutes, from time to time pour the juice over the chicken with a cup. After cooked let it cool and cut in pieces.

Green rice:

Ingredients:

- 2 cups of rice

- 3 cups of water

- 1 cup of coriander

- 1/4 cup of celery

- 1/4 cup of chili

- 30 g of olive oil

- salt

Procedure: In a pot, warm the oil and Styr-fry the rice. Once rice is brown, add salt and then water. Add the coriander, celery and chilies without seeds and milled. Move immediately so the flavor will stick to the rice. Let it boil. Cover and cook it for 20 minutes with low fire.

Nutritional facts (chicken and rice): Energy 524 kcal, protein 34 g, total fat 15 g, cholesterol 136 mg, carbohydrates 40 g, fiber 5.8 and sodium 385 mg.

53.   Green cause of coriander

Ingredients:

- 1 kg of potatoes

- 1 bundle of coriander

- 1 bundle of spinach

- 1 ½ avocado

- 2 cans of tuna on water

- salt and pepper

- ginger powder

- 5 spoons of olive oil

- aluminum foil

- red pepper cut in julienne style to decorate

Mayonnaise of potato:

Ingredients:

- 2 potatoes

- 1 carrot

- 1/2 cup of milk

- 1/2 cup of olive oil

- salt

Procedure: Dry the coriander leaves and mix in the blender with olive oil and boiled spinach leaves. Reserve it aside. Boil the potatoes in cold water with salt, once they are cooked and warm, mill with a press and add the spinach oil and coriander. Add salt and pepper. Cut the avocado in slices on the thin side and dress with salt, pepper and lemon juice. Prepare the potato mayonnaise. Cook the potatoes and carrots; mix with milk, oil and salt in the blender. Foil a fount of 10x35 cm with aluminum foil and pour oil over it. Now build a layer of 3 cm of potato, spinach and coriander, and then add a layer of potato mayonnaise. Follow it with a layer of avocado and another of potato mayonnaise. To finish add a layer of tuna and then one final of potato mayonnaise. To serve decorate with avocado, tuna and red pepper.

Nutritional facts: Energy 235 kcal, proteins 11 g, total fat 8.8 g, cholesterol 17.1 mg, carbohydrate 30.3 g, fiber 6.2 g and sodium 323 mg.

54. Ceviche of mushrooms and artichokes (for 4 people)

Ingredients:

- 300 g of mushrooms

- 3 bottoms of big artichokes

- 1/2 little spoon of milled pepper

- 2 chilies cut in julienne style

- 1/2 spoon of parsley

- 1/2 spoon of coriander

- 2 spoons of olive oil

- 1/2 purple onion

- lemon juice

- lettuce leaves to decorate

Procedure: Clean and wash the artichoke bottoms. Put them with water and salt in a pot, add a little lemon juice and boil until the artichokes are soft. Drain, let it cool and cut in strips. Clean the mushrooms with absorbent paper and cut them in little strips. Put the mushrooms and the artichoke together. Dress the mixture with salt, pepper, chili, coriander and parsley. Mix it really good. Add the lemon juice, olive oil and onions. Move and serve.

Nutritional facts: Energy 85.3 kcal, protein 3.6 g, total fat 3.4 g, cholesterol 0 mg, carbohydrates 13.2 g, fiber 6.6 g and sodium 281 mg.

55. Roast beef with vegetables sauce (for 6 people)

Ingredients:

- 1 kg of beef without fat (steak)

- 1 onion cut in squares

- 2 carrots cut in squares

- 1 garlic teeth

- chicken consommé

- salt, pepper and laurel leaves

- 1 spoon of corn flour

Procedure: Fry the onions, garlic and carrots in a pot until they are brown. Grill the beef until is brown on every side. Put the beef on the top and the vegetables over them in order not to get burned at the bottom. Dress with salt, pepper and laurel. Add the chicken consommé until it covers the half of the beef. Cover and let it cook for one hour. Take out the beef and mix the vegetables in the blender. If the mixture is too liquid add the corn flour to add consistency. Cut the beef on slices and serve with the vegetable sauce. For a vegetable consommé put in a pot celery, carrots, onion and pepper; cover with water, dress with salt and pepper and let it boil until the vegetables are cooked and then drain.

Nutritional facts: Energy 164 kcal, proteins 23.4 g, total fat 4.15 g, cholesterol 68 mg, carbohydrates 5.92, fiber 0.7 g and sodium 281 mg.

56. Chicken salmagundi with watercress and avocado (for 6 people)

Ingredients:

- 1 boiled chicken chest

- 2 spoons of lemon juice

- salt and pepper

- 3 spoons of olive oil

- 2 cups of purple lettuce

- 2 cups of green lettuce

- 2 cups of watercress

- 1 onion cut in julienne style

- 1/2 avocado cut in cubes

- 3 eggs cut by the half

Procedure: Cut the chicken in little pieces. In a bowl mix lemon juice, salt and pepper, and add a little olive oil meanwhile mixing. Check salt and reserve. In a salad pot put the lettuces, watercress, onion, avocado and chicken. Pour the dressing and mix. Add the egg on top and let the mixture rest for 15 minutes. Now is ready to serve.

Nutritional facts: energy 164 kcal, protein 13.8 g, total fat 11 g, cholesterol 64.3 mg, carbohydrates 3.1 g, fiber 2.5 g and sodium 252 mg.

57.   Chicken creole soup

Ingredients:

- 2 cooked chicken chest

- 2 slices of bread

- 2 cups of lactose free milk

- 1 cup of onion cut in squares

- 1 ½ cup of chicken consommé

- 1 spoon of chili

- 1 white egg

- salt and pepper

- 2 boiled eggs and parsley to decorate

Procedure: Put the bread in a bowl with the milk and let it soak for 15 minutes. Mix together in the blender. Cut the chicken in thin slices. In a pot, brown the onions with a little chicken consommé. Once it's brown add the chili, consommé, bread, salt and pepper. Let it cook for 5 minutes, add the chicken. Serve in a baking fount. Add the white egg and take it to the oven for 10 minutes. Decorate with the boiled eggs and parsley. Add salad to join.

Nutritional facts: Energy 191 kcal, proteins 23.4 g, total fat 4.9 , cholesterol 99 mg, carbohydrates 12.4 g, fiber 1 g and sodium 386 mg.

58. Italian squash soup (for 6 people)

Ingredients:

- 1 liter of chicken consommé

- 3 Italian squash with skin

Procedure: In a pot for oven, boil the chicken consommé. Wash the squash, separate the hard sides and cut the rest in big slices with skin. Cook the squash in the consommé for 10 minutes. Mix together in a blender. Serve warm. Beware that you should only mix with a wood spoon.

Nutritional facts: Energy 30 kcal, protein 1.6 g, total fat 2 g, cholesterol 26.3 mg, carbohydrates 2.1 g, fiber 1 g and sodium 241 mg.

59.   Oriental salad (for 8 people)

Ingredients:

- 2 cups of boiled chicken in cubes
- 4 cups of lettuce
- 2 cups of boiled prawns in cubes
- 1 carrot
- 4 chives
- 1 spoon of sesame seeds

Dressing:

- 6 spoons of olive oil
- 5 spoons of white vinegar
- 1 spoon of sugar
- 1/2 spoon of lemon juice
- 1/2 spoon of ginger powder
- 1/2 spoon of salt

Procedure: Put all the vegetables together in a bowl. In a pan put the chicken and the prawns and sauté. Add it to the vegetables and mix. Pour the dressing while serving.

Nutritional facts: Energy 153 kcal, proteins 5.5 g, total fat 2.9 g, cholesterol 95.2 mg, carbohydrates 23.7 g, fiber 0.6 g and sodium 80.2 mg.

60.   California salad and chicken schnitzel (for 6 people)

Ingredients:

- 1 lettuce cut in strips

- 4 cups of boiled spinach

- 2 grated carrots

- 1 cup of tomatoes cut in squares

- 1 celery stick

- 1/2 cup of raisins

- 1/2 cup of toasted almonds

- 2 spoons of sesame seed

Dressing:

- 3 spoons of olive oil

- 2 spoons of vinegar

- 2 spoons of palm honey

- orange juice

- salt and milled pepper

Chicken schnitzel:

- 600 g of chicken filet

- salt and oregano

Procedure: Put all the vegetables together. Mix the ingredients of the dressing. Serve in individual dishes. Grill the chicken schnitzel with a little oil and dress with salt and pepper.

Nutritional facts (salad and chicken): Energy 233 kcal, protein 6 g, total fat 36.9 g, cholesterol 86.9 mg, carbohydrates 7.7 g, fiber 2.5 g and sodium 319 mg.

61. Tangerine, lactose free milk with coffee, toasted bread with scrambled eggs

Ingredients:

- 3 tangerines
- 1 cup of lactose free milk
- 2 spoons of coffee
- 2 slices of toasted bread
- 2 eggs
- olive oil

Procedure: Three tangerines, one cup of lactose free milk with coffee, two slices of toasted bread with scrambled eggs, eggs fried on olive oil.

Nutritional facts: Energy 344 kcal, protein 15.9 g, total fat 8.2 g, cholesterol 229 mg, carbohydrates 43.2 g, fiber 2.8 g and sodium 394 mg.

62.   Melon, tea with lactose free milk, toasted bread with low calories jam

Ingredients:

- 1 cup of melon cut on squares
- 1/2 cup of lactose free milk
- 1/2 cup of tea
- 2 toasted bread
- 3 slices of cheese
- 3 spoons of low calories jam

Procedure: A cup of melon cut on little squares, one big cup of lactose free milk with tea, two toasted bread with cheese and low calories jam.

Nutritional facts: Energy 242 kcal, proteins 14.8 g, total at 3.6 g, cholesterol 8.1 mg, carbohydrates 38.6 g, fiber 2.9 g and sodium 357.4 mg.

63. Milk with coffee, fruit salad and dried fruits

Ingredients:

- 1 glass of lactose free milk

- 2 spoons of coffee

- 1/2 orange

- 1/2 apple

- 5 raisins

- 5 almonds

- 2 nuts

Procedure: Lactose free milk mixed with coffee. Put in a bowl half orange, half apple, 5 raisins, 5 almonds and two nuts.

Nutritional facts: Energy 263 kcal, protein 9.5 g, total fat 10.2 g, cholesterol 16 mg, carbohydrates 28.3 g, fiber 3.6 g and sodium 101 mg.

64.   Tea with lactose-free milk, whole meal bread and two scrambled eggs

Ingredients:

- 1/2 cup of tea

- 1/2 cup of lactose-free milk

- 1 slice of whole meal bread

- 2 eggs

- olive oil

Procedure: Serve one cup of tea with lactose-free milk. One slice of whole meal bread with two scrambled eggs, eggs fried with olive oil.

Nutritional facts: Energy 342 kcal, protein 21.5 g, total fat 8.9 g, cholesterol 215.6 mg, carbohydrates 46.1 g, fiber 5.9 g and sodium 673 mg.

JUICES

1.   Pineapple Spinach Juice

Ingredients:

1 cup of pineapple, chunked

1 cup of spinach, chopped

1 cup of cherries, pitted

1 whole lemon, peeled

¼ tsp of cinnamon, ground

1 oz of water

Preparation:

Using a sharp paring knife, cut the top of the pineapple. Gently remove all hard skin and slice it into thin slices. Fill the measuring cup and reserve the rest for later.

Rinse the spinach thoroughly under cold running water. Drain and chop into small pieces. Set aside.

Place the cherries in a medium colander. Rinse well under cold running water and remove the stems, if any. Cut each in half and remove the pits. Fill the measuring cup and reserve the rest in the refrigerator.

Peel the lemon and cut lengthwise in half. Set aside.

Now, combine pineapple, spinach, cherries, and lemon in a juicer and process until juiced. Transfer to a serving glass and stir in the water.

Add some crushed ice and serve immediately.

Nutrition information per serving: Kcal: 196, Protein: 9.2g, Carbs: 59.3g, Fats: 1.5g

2. Cantaloupe Cucumber Juice

Ingredients:

1 cup of cantaloupe, peeled and chopped

1 large cucumber

1 cup of avocado, peeled and pitted

1 large lemon, peeled

Preparation:

Cut the cantaloupe in half. Scoop out the seeds and flesh. Cut two wedges and peel them. Chop into chunks and set aside. Reserve the rest of the cantaloupe in a refrigerator.

Wash the cucumber and cut into thick slices. Set aside.

Peel the avocado and cut in half. Remove the pit and cut into chunks. Set aside.

Peel the lemon and cut in half. Set aside.

Now, process cantaloupe, cucumber, avocado, and lemon in a juicer.

Transfer to serving glasses and add some water to adjust the thickness, if needed.

Add some ice and serve immediately.

Nutritional information per serving: Kcal: 292, Protein: 6.8g, Carbs: 41.5g, Fats: 22.2g

3.   Parsnip Carrot Juice

Ingredients:

1 cup of parsnip, sliced

1 large carrot, sliced

1 cup of cauliflower, chopped

1 cup of fennel, trimmed and chopped

1 whole lime, peeled

Preparation:

Wash and peel the parsnip and carrot. Cut into thin slices and fill the measuring cup. Reserve the rest for later.

Wash the cauliflower and trim off the outer leaves. Cut into small pieces and fill the measuring cup. Reserve the rest for later.

Trim off the fennel stalks and outer wilted layers. Wash and chop the fennel into bite-sized pieces. Fill the measuring cup and reserve the rest for later. Set aside.

Peel the lime and cut lengthwise in half. Set aside.

Now, combine parsnip, carrot, cauliflower, fennel, and lime in a juicer. Process until well juiced.

Transfer to a serving glass and refrigerate for 10 minutes before serving.

Add some turmeric or ginger for some extra taste. However, it's optional.

Nutrition information per serving: Kcal: 141, Protein: 5.6g, Carbs: 46.2g, Fats: 1.1g

4. Grapefruit Broccoli Juice

Ingredients:

1 large grapefruit, peeled

1 cup of broccoli

1 large apricot, pitted

1 large banana

Preparation:

Peel the grapefruit and cut into bite-sized pieces. Set aside.

Place the broccoli in a colander and wash under cold running water. Chop into small pieces and set aside.

Wash the apricot and cut in half. Remove the pit and cut into small pieces. Set aside.

Peel the banana and cut into small chunks. Set aside.

Now, process grapefruit, broccoli, apricot, and banana in a juicer. Transfer to serving glasses and refrigerate for 30 minutes before serving.

Nutritional information per serving: Kcal: 229, Protein: 6.5g, Carbs: 67.2g, Fats: 1.3g

5.   Brussels Sprout Parsley Juice

Ingredients:

1 cup of Brussels sprouts, chopped

1 cup of parsley, chopped

2 whole leeks, chopped

2 whole kiwis, chopped

A handful of spinach, chopped

½ cup of water

Preparation:

Wash the Brussels sprouts and trim off the outer leaves. Cut in half and set aside.

Wash the parsley in a colander under cold running water and set aside.

Wash the leeks and chop into small pieces. Set aside.

Peel the kiwis and cut in half. Set aside.

Wash the spinach thoroughly and set aside.

Now, process Brussels sprouts, parsley, leeks, kiwis, and spinach in a juicer. Transfer to serving glasses and stir in the water.

Refrigerate for 5 minutes before serving.

Nutritional information per serving: Kcal: 207, Protein: 9.8g, Carbs: 58.1g, Fats: 2.1g

6.   Orange Carrot Juice

Ingredients:

1 large orange, peeled

1 large carrot, sliced

1 cup of crookneck squash, cubed

1 whole lemon, peeled

1 cup of cucumber, sliced

¼ tsp of turmeric, ground

Preparation:

Peel the orange and divide into wedges. Cut each wedge in half and set aside.

Wash and peel the carrot. Cut into thin slices and set aside.

Wash the squash and chop into small cubes. Fill the measuring cup and reserve the rest in the refrigerator. Set aside.

Peel the lemon and cut lengthwise in half. Set aside.

Wash the cucumber and cut into thin slices. Fill the measuring cup and reserve the rest for later.

Now, combine orange, carrot, squash, lemon, and cucumber in a juicer and process until juiced. Transfer to a serving glass and stir in the turmeric.

Add some crushed ice and serve immediately.

Nutrition information per serving: Kcal: 127, Protein: 4.6g, Carbs: 40.7g, Fats: 0.9g

7.   Cucumber Artichoke Juice

Ingredients:

1 cup of turnip greens

1 large cucumber

1 large artichoke head

5 large asparagus spears

Preparation:

Wash the cucumber and cut into thick slices. Set aside.

Using a sharp knife, trim off the outer leave of the artichoke. Cut into small pieces and set aside.

Wash the turnip greens and roughly chop it using hands. Set aside.

Wash the asparagus spears and trim off the woody ends. Cut into small pieces and set aside.

Now, process cucumber, artichoke, turnip greens, and asparagus in a juicer.

Transfer to serving glasses and add few ice cubes before serving.

Nutritional information per serving: Kcal: 101, Protein: 10.1g, Carbs: 35.8g, Fats: 0.8g

8.   Mango Apricot Juice

Ingredients:

1 cup of mango, chunked

3 whole apricots, chopped

1 cup of blackberries

1 cup of fresh spinach, torn

1 whole lime, peeled

Preparation:

Peel the mango and cut into small chunks. Fill the measuring cup and reserve the rest for later. Set aside.

Wash the apricots and cut in half. Remove the pits and chop into small pieces. Set aside.

Rinse the blackberries using a large colander. Drain and set aside.

Rinse the spinach thoroughly under cold running water. Drain and torn into small pieces. Set aside.

Peel the lime and cut lengthwise in half. Set aside.

Now, combine mango, apricots, blackberries, spinach, and lime in a juicer. Process until juiced. Transfer to a serving glass and refrigerate for 10 minutes before serving.

Enjoy!

Nutrition information per serving: Kcal: 201, Protein: 11.1g, Carbs: 61.5g, Fats: 2.6g

9.   Celery Mint Juice

Ingredients:

5 small celery stalks

¼ cup od fresh mint

¼ cup of fresh spinach

1 large lime, peeled

3 oz of coconut water

Preparation:

Wash the celery stalks and chop into small pieces. Set aside.

Combine mint and spinach in a large colander. Wash thoroughly under cold running water and drain. Torn into small pieces and set aside.

Peel the lime and cut in half. Set aside.

Combine lime, celery, spinach, and mint in a juicer and process until juiced.

Transfer to serving glasses and stir in coconut water. Refrigerate for 20 minutes before use.

Nutritional information per serving: Kcal: 45, Protein: 2.2g, Carbs: 16.8g, Fats: 1.6g

10. Lemon Pepper Juice

Ingredients:

1 large lemon, peeled

½ red bell pepper, seeded

½ yellow bell pepper, seeded

1 green apple, cored

2 tbsp of chia seeds

Preparation:

Peel the lemon and cut lengthwise in half. Place it in a bowl and set aside.

Wash the bell pepper and cut in half. Remove the seeds and cut one-half of each in a bowl. Reserve the rest for some other juice.

Wash the apple and remove the core. Cut into bite-sized pieces and set aside.

Now, process lemon, bell peppers, and apple in a juicer. Transfer to serving glasses and stir in the chia seeds. Refrigerate for 15 minutes and stir again. Add some water to adjust the thickness, if needed.

Nutritional information per serving: Kcal: 136, Protein: 4.3g, Carbs: 31.2g, Fats: 6.1g

11. Pineapple Lemon Juice

Ingredients:

1 cup of pineapple, peeled

½ large lemon, peeled

1 cup of watermelon, peeled and seeded

½ tsp of ginger, ground

Preparation:

Cut the top of the pineapple using a sharp paring knife. Gently remove all hard skin and slice it into thin slices. Fill the measuring cup and reserve the rest for later.

Peel the lemon and cut lentghwise in half. Reserve one half in the refrigerator for later. Set aside.

Now, combine all ingredients in a juicer and process until juiced.

Transfer to serving glasses and add few ice cubes. Serve immediately!

Nutritional information per serving: Kcal: 41, Protein: 1.4g, Carbs: 10.2g, Fats: 0.1g

12. Cucumber Pear Juice

Ingredients:

2 large cucumbers

1 large pear, cored

1 cup of black grapes

1 lime, peeled

Preparation:

Wash the cucumbers and cut into thin slices. Set aside.

Wash the pear and cut in half. Remove the core and chop into bite-sized pieces. Set aside.

Wash the grapes and remove the pit. Set aside.

Peel the lime and cut lengthwise in half. Set aside.

Now, combine cucumbers, pear, grapes, and lime in a juicer and process until juiced.

Transfer to serving glasses and refrigerate for 5 minutes before serving.

Nutritional information per serving: Kcal: 113, Protein: 18.3g, Carbs: 31.3g, Fats: 0.1g

13.   Cabbage Lemon Juice

Ingredients:

1 cup of green cabbage

1 large lemon, peeled

A handful of spinach

1 medium-sized artichoke head

1 large cucumber

Preparation:

Wash the cabbage and spinach thoroughly and torn with hands. Set aside.

Peel the lemon and cut lengthwise in half. Set aside.

Using a sharp knife, trim off the outer leave of the artichoke. Cut into small pieces and set aside.

Wash the cucumber and cut into thick slices. Set aside.

Process, cabbage, lemon, spinach, cucumber, and artichoke in a juicer.

Transfer to serving glasses and add some ice.

Nutritional information per serving: Kcal: 99, Protein: 8.8g, Carbs: 36.4g, Fats: 0.9g

14.   Kale Lettuce Juice

Ingredients:

1 cup of fresh kale

1 cup of Romaine lettuce

1 cup of Swiss chard

1 large tomato

1 large fennel bulb

1 cup of collard greens

Preparation:

Wash the kale, lettuce, Swiss chard, and collard greens thoroughly under cold running water. Torn with hands and set aside. Wash the tomato and chop into quarters. Set aside.

Wash the fennel bulb and trim off the wilted outer layers. Cut into small chunks and set aside. Now, process kale, lettuce, Swiss chard, tomato, fennel and collard greens in a juicer. Transfer to serving glasses and refrigerate for 15 minutes before serving.

Nutritional information per serving: Kcal: 106, Protein: 9.7g, Carbs: 34.8g, Fats: 1.8g

15.   Artichoke Potato Juice

Ingredients:

1 large artichoke head

1 cup of sweet potatoes, cubed

1 large bunch of spinach

1 cup of turnip greens, chopped

1 cup of basil, chopped

2 oz of water

¼ tsp of Himalayan salt

Preparation:

Trim off the outer leaves of the artichoke using a sharp knife. Cut into bite-sized pieces and set aside.

Peel the sweet potato and cut into chunks. Set aside.

Combine spinach, turnip greens, and basil in a colander and wash under cold running water. Drain and chop it roughly with your hands and set aside.

Now, process artichoke, sweet potato, spinach, turnip greens, and basil in a juicer. Transfer to serving glasses and stir in the water and Himalayan salt.

Add some ice and serve immediately.

Nutritional information per serving: Kcal: 202, Protein: 18.6g, Carbs: 60.7g, Fats: 1.9g

16.   Green Lemon Apple Juice

Ingredients:

1 whole lemon, peeled

2 large green apples, cored

½ cup of fresh kale

1 large pear, cored

Preparation:

Peel the lemon and cut lengthwise in half. Set aside.

Wash the apple and cut in half. Remove the cores and chop into bite-sized pieces. Set aside.

Wash the kale thoroughly under cold running water. Drain and torn into small pieces. Set aside.

Wash the pear and cut in half. Remove the core and chop into small pieces. Set aside.

Now, combine all lemon, apples, kale, and pear in a juicer and process until juiced.

Transfer to serving glasses and add few ice cubes before serving.

Nutritional information per serving: Kcal: 120, Protein: 3.2g, Carbs: 62.5g, Fats: 1.2g

17.   Broccoli Carrot Juice

Ingredients:

½ cup of fresh broccoli, chopped

3 large carrots

2 large oranges, peeled

4 collard green leaves

4 fresh kale leaves

1 garlic clove, peeled

Preparation:

Wash the broccoli thoroughly and trim off the outer layers. Chop into small pieces and reserve the rest for later. Set aside.

Wash the carrots and chop into small pieces.

Peel the oranges and divide into wedges. Set aside.

Rinse the collard greens under cold running water and drain. Torn into small pieces and set aside.

Now, combine broccoli, carrots, oranges, and collard greens in a juicer and process until juiced.

Transfer to serving glasses and serve immediately.

Nutritional information per serving: Kcal: 171, Protein: 9.2g, Carbs: 43.3g, Fats: 2.3g

18.   Broccoli Cucumber Juice

Ingredients:

1 cup of broccoli, chopped

1 large cucumber

1 cup of avocado, chopped

1 large lemon, peeled

1 large lime, peeled

1 oz of water

Preparation:

Wash the broccoli and chop into small pieces. Set aside.

Wash the cucumber and cut in thick slices. Set aside.

Peel the avocado and cut in half. Remove the pit and cut into chunks. Set aside.

Peel the lemon and lime. Cut lengthwise in half. Set aside.

Now, process broccoli, cucumber, avocado, lemon, and lime in a juicer. Transfer to serving glasses and stir in the water. Add some ice and serve immediately.

Nutritional information per serving: Kcal: 281, Protein: 8.3g, Carbs: 38.8g, Fats: 22.8g

19.   Beet Turmeric Juice

Ingredients:

1 cup of beet greens, torn

¼ tsp of turmeric powder, ground

2 cups of parsley, torn

1 whole cucumber, sliced

1 cup of celery, chopped

1 whole leek, chopped

¼ tsp of cumin, ground

Preparation:

Combine beet greens and parsley in a large colander. Rinse well under cold running water and drain. Torn into small pieces and set aside.

Wash the cucumber and cut into thin slices. Set aside.

Wash the celery and chop into small pieces. Fill the measuring cup and reserve the rest in the refrigerator. Set aside.

Wash the leek and chop into bite-sized pieces. Set aside.

Now, combine parsley, beet greens, cucumber, celery, and leek in a juicer and process until juiced. Transfer to a serving glass and stir in the turmeric and cumin.

Serve immediately.

Nutrition information per serving: Kcal: 127, Protein: 8.4g, Carbs: 35.7g, Fats: 1.7g

20.   Cucumber Pineapple Juice

Ingredients:

1 large cucumber

1 cup of pineapple, chopped

3 celery stalks

½ cup of fresh spinach

¼ tsp of ginger, ground

¼ tsp of turmeric, ground

Preparation:

Wash the cucumber and cut into thin slices. Set aside.

Cut the top of the pineapple using a sharp paring knife. Gently remove all hard skin and slice it into thin slices. Fill the measuring cup and reserve the rest for later.

Wash the celery and cut into small pieces. Set aside.

Rinse the spinach thoroughly under cold running water and drain. Torn into small pieces and set aside.

Now, combine cucumber, pineapple, celery, and spinach in a juicer and process until juiced.

Transfer to serving glasses and stir in the turmeric and ginger.

Serve immediately.

Nutritional information per serving: Kcal: 109, Protein: 3.3g, Carbs: 61.2g, Fats: 1.3g

21.   Orange Cucumber Juice

Ingredients:

1 cup of broccoli, chopped

2 large oranges, peeled

1 large cucumber, peeled

1 large carrot

Preparation:

Wash the broccoli and trim off the outer leaves. Cut into small pieces and fill the measuring cup. Reserve the rest in the refrigerator.

Peel the oranges and divide into wedges. Set aside.

Wash the cucumber and cut into thin slices. Set aside.

Now, combine broccoli, oranges, cucumber, and carrot in a juicer and process until juiced.

Transfer to serving glasses and add few ice cubes.

Serve immediately!

Nutritional information per serving: Kcal: 68, Protein: 2.3g, Carbs: 19.7g, Fats: 0.1g

22.   Apple Ginger Juice

Ingredients:

1 large Granny Smith's apple, cored and chopped

1 small ginger knob, peeled

1 cup of celery, chopped

1 cup of fresh mint, torn

¼ tsp of liquid honey

1 oz of water

Preparation:

Wash the apple and cut lengthwise in half. Remove the core and cut into bite-sized pieces. Set aside.

Peel the ginger knob and chop into small pieces. Set aside.

Wash the celery and chop into small pieces. Fill the measuring cup and reserve the rest for later.

Rinse the mint thoroughly under cold running water. Dran and torn into small pieces.

Now, combine apple, ginger, celery, and mint in a juicer and process until well juiced. Transfer to a serving glass and stir in the honey and water.

Refrigerate for 5 minutes before serving.

Enjoy!

Nutrition information per serving: Kcal: 121, Protein: 2.6g, Carbs: 35.8g, Fats: 0.8g

23.   Spring Onion Pepper Juice

Ingredients:

1 medium-sized spring onion

1 large bell pepper, seeded

1 cup of cherry tomatoes

1 garlic clove, peeled

¼ tsp of Cayenne pepper, ground

¼ tsp of salt

A handful of fresh cilantro

Preparation:

Wash the spring onion and chop into small pieces. Set aside.

Wash the bell pepper and cut in half. Remove the seeds and chop into small pieces. Set aside.

Wash the cilantro thoroughly and torn with hands. Set aside.

Wash the cherry tomatoes and place them in a bowl. Cut in half and reserve the juice while cutting. Set aside.

Peel the garlic and set aside.

Now, process spring onion, bell pepper, cilantro, tomatoes, and garlic in a juicer.

Transfer to serving glasses and stir in Cayenne pepper and salt.

Refrigerate for 5 minutes and serve.

Nutritional information per serving: Kcal: 41, Protein: 2.8g, Carbs: 11.5g, Fats: 0.6g

24.   Grape Apple Juice

Ingredients:

1 cup of green grapes

1 Granny Smith apple, cored

3 large carrots

1 large lemon, peeled

A handful of spinach

2 oz of water

Preparation:

Wash the grapes and set aside.

Wash the apple and remove the core. Cut into bite-sized pieces and set aside.

Wash the carrots and cut into thick slices. Set aside.

Peel the lemon and cut lengthwise in half. Set aside.

Wash the spinach thoroughly under cold running water. Roughly chop it and set aside.

Now, combine grapes, apple, carrots, lemon, and spinach in a juicer and process until juiced. Transfer to serving glasses and stir in the water.

Refrigerate for 10 minutes before serving.

Enjoy!

Nutritional information per serving: Kcal: 208, Protein: 1.4g, Carbs: 62.6g, Fats: 1.4g

25.   Broccoli Carrot Juice

Ingredients:

1 cup of fresh broccoli

4 large carrots

1 large green apple, cored

1 tsp of ginger root

2 cups of cauliflower, chopped

Preparation:

Wash the broccoli and trim off the outer leaves. Cut into small pieces and fill the measuring cups. Reserve the rest in the refrigerator.

Wash the carrots and cut into thin slices. Set aside.

Wash the apple and cut in half. Remove the core and cut into bite-sized pieces. Set aside.

Peel the ginger root and set aside.

Wash the cauliflower and trim off the outer leaves. Chop into small pieces and set aside.

Now, combine broccoli, carrots, apple, ginger, and cauliflower in a juicer and process until juiced.

Transfer to serving glasses and optionally, garnish with mint.

Enjoy!

Nutritional information per serving: Kcal: 136, Protein: 6.3g, Carbs: 42.8g, Fats: 1.2g

26.   Apple Spinach Juice

Ingredients:

1 large apple, cored

1 cup of fresh spinach

1 tbsp of chia seeds

¼ tsp of cinnamon, ground

Preparation:

Wash the apple and cut in half. Remove the core and cut into bite-sized pieces. Set aside.

Wash the spinach thoroughly under cold running water.Drain and torn into small pieces. Set aside.

Now, combine apple, spinach, and chia in a juicer and process until juiced.

Transfer to serving glasses and stir in the cinnamon.

Refrigerate for 10 minutes and serve.

Nutritional information per serving: Kcal: 121, Protein: 4.3g, Carbs: 27.8g, Fats: 5.3g

27.   Pear Carrot Juice

Ingredients:

1 large pear, cored

3 large carrots

1 medium-sized cucumber

1 large lemon, peeled

¼ cup of fresh mint

½ cup of broccoli

½ tsp of ginger, ground

½ tsp of green tea powder

2 oz of water

Preparation:

Wash the pear and cut in half. Remove the core and chop into small pieces. Set aside.

Wash the carrots and cucumber. Cut into thin slices and set aside.

Peel the lemon and cut lengthwise in half. Set aside.

Combine pear, carrots, cucumber, lemon, mint, ginger, and

broccoli in a juicer and process until juiced.

Mix water with green tea in a serving glasses and add juice.

Mix with a spoon and add few ice cubes. Serve immediately.

Nutritional information per serving: Kcal: 141, Protein: 5.5g, Carbs: 45.7g, Fats: 0.9g

28.   Watercress Pumpkin Juice

Ingredients:

1 cup of watercress, chopped

1 cup of pumpkin, chopped

1 cup of cherry tomatoes, halved

1 cup of collard greens, chopped

1 large cucumber

Preparation:

Combine watercress and collard greens in a colander and wash thoroughly. Torn with hands and set aside.

Peel the pumpkin and cut in half. Scoop out the seeds using a spoon. Cut one large wedge and peel it. Cut into small chunks and set aside. Reserve the rest for later.

Wash the tomatoes and place them in a bowl. Cut in half and reserve the juice in the bowl while cutting. Set aside.

Wash the cucumber and cut into thick slices. Set aside.

Now, process watercress, collard greens, pumpkin, tomatoes, and cucumber in a juicer. Transfer to serving glasses and stir in the reserved tomato juice. Add some ice before serving.

Enjoy!

Nutritional information per serving: Kcal: 96, Protein: 6.4g, Carbs: 27.4g, Fats: 1g

29.   Zucchini Asparagus Juice

Ingredients:

2 medium-sized zucchini, sliced

6 medium asparagus stalks, trimmed and chopped

3 Roma tomatoes, chopped

4 large carrots, sliced

Preparation:

Wash the zucchini and cut into thin slices. Set aside.

Wash the asparagus and trim off the woody ends. cut into small pieces. Set aside.

Wash the tomatoes and cut into small pieces. Make sure to reserve the juices while cutting.

Wash the carrots and cut into thin slices. Set aside.

Now, combine all ingredients in a juicer and process until juiced.

Transfer to serving glasses and enjoy immediately.

Nutritional information per serving: Kcal: 92, Protein: 5.4g, Carbs: 27.3g, Fats: 0.9g

30.   Celery Apple Juice

Ingredients:

3 celery stalks

1 large green apple, cored

1 large lemon, peeled

½ cup of cilantro

½ tsp of ginger, ground

Preparation:

Wash the celery and chop into small pieces. Set aside.

Wash the apple and cut in half. Remove the core and cut into small pieces. Set aside.

Peel the lemon and cut lengthwise in half. Set aside.

Now, combine celery, apple, lemon, and cilantro in a juicer. Process until juiced. Transfer to serving glasses and stir in the ginger.

Add few ice cubes and serve immediately.

Nutritional information per serving: Kcal: 73, Protein: 2.2g, Carbs: 26.7g, Fats: 0.1g

31.   Chia Carrot Juice

Ingredients:

3 large carrots

2 large apples, cored

½ tsp of ginger, ground

1 tbsp of chia seeds

Preparation:

Wash the carrots and cut into thin slices. Set aside.

Wash the apples and cut in half. Remove the core and cut into bite-sized pieces. Set aside.

Now, combine carrots, apples, and ginger in a juicer and process until juiced.

Transfer to serving glasses and stir in the chia seeds. Add few ice cubes and enjoy!

Nutritional information per serving: Kcal: 177, Protein: 3.2g, Carbs: 28.4g, Fats: 4.6g

32.   Kale Apple Juice

Ingredients:

1 medium fennel

½ cup of fresh kale

1 large green apple, cored

4 tangerines, peeled

Preparation:

Wash the kale thoroughly under cold running water. Drain and set aside.

Wash the apple and cut in half. Remove the core and cut into bite-sized pieces. Set aside. Peel the tangerines and divide into wedges. Set aside.

Trim off the outside layers of the fennel. Wash it and cut into bite-sized pieces. Set aside. Now, combine kale, apple, tangerines, and fennel in a juicer and process until juiced.

Transfer to serving glasses and add few ice cubes or refrigerate before use.

Nutritional information per serving: Kcal: 121, Protein: 4.3g, Carbs: 31.3g, Fats: 1.3g

33.   Lime Cucumber Juice

Ingredients:

1 large lime, peeled

1 large cucumber

½ cup of fresh kale

1 celery stalk

1 small jalapeno pepper, seeded

Preparation:

Peel the lime and cut lengthwise in half. Set aside.

Wash the cucumber and cut into thin slices. Set aside.

Rinse the kale thoroughly under cold running water. Drain and set aside. Wash the celery and chop it into small pieces. Set aside.

Now, combine lime, cucumber, kale, and celery in a juicer and process until juiced. Add coconut water if it is too spicy.

Transfer to serving glasses and add a few ice cubes. Serve immediately.

Nutritional information per serving: Kcal: 171, Protein: 3.2g, Carbs: 47.3g, Fats: 1.3g

34.   Pomegranate Pumpkin Juice

Ingredients:

1 cup of pomegranate seeds

1 cup of pumpkin, cubed

1 medium-sized orange, peeled

3 whole plums, pitted and chopped

¼ tsp of ginger, ground

1 oz of water

Preparation:

Cut the top of the pomegranate fruit using a sharp paring knife. Slice down to each of the white membranes inside of the fruit. Pop the seeds into a measuring cup and set aside.

Cut the top of a pumpkin. Cut lengthwise in half and then scrape out the seeds. Cut one large wedge and peel it. Cut into small cubes and fill the measuring cup. Reserve the rest in the refrigerator.

Wash the plums and cut into halves. Remove the pits and chop into small pieces.Set aside.

Peel the orange and divide into wedges. Cut each wedge in

half and set aside.

Now, combine pomegranate, pumpkin, plums, and orange in a juicer. Process until juiced. Transfer to a serving glass and stir in the ginger and water.

Refrigerate for 5 minutes before serving.

Enjoy!

Nutrition information per serving: Kcal: 214, Protein: 5.2g, Carbs: 61.8g, Fats: 1.8g

35.   Kiwi Cucumber Juice

Ingredients:

2 kiwis, peeled

1 large cucumber

1 cup of fresh strawberries

1 whole lime, peeled

2 tbsp of fresh mint

Preparation:

Peel the kiwis and cut in half. Set aside.

Wash the cucumber and cut into thin slices. Set aside.

Wash the strawberries and remove the top stems, if any. Cut into small pieces and set aside. Peel the lime and cut lengthwise in half. Set aside.

Now, combine kiwis, cucumber, strawberries, lime and mint in a juicer and process until juiced.

Transfer to serving glasses and refrigerate for a while until use.

Nutritional information per serving: Kcal: 91, Protein: 3.1g, Carbs: 29.9g, Fats: 0.9g

36.   Beet Fennel Juice

Ingredients:

1 cup of beets, chopped

1 cup of fennel, sliced

2 large tomatoes, peeled

1 tbsp of fresh mint, chopped

1 cup of red leaf lettuce, shredded

½ tsp of ginger, ground

Preparation:

Wash the beets and trim off the green ends. Cut into small pieces and set aside.

Wash the fennel bulb and trim off the wilted outer layers. Cut into small chunks and set aside.

Wash the tomatoes and place them in a bowl. Cut into quarters and reserve the juice while cutting.

Wash the lettuce thoroughly and torn with hands. Set aside.

Now, combine beets, fennel, tomatoes, mint, and lettuce in a juicer and process until juiced.

Transfer to serving glasses and stir in the ground ginger.

Refrigerate for 10 minutes before serving.

Nutritional information per serving: Kcal: 111, Protein: 6.9g, Carbs: 34.8g, Fats: 1.2g

37.   Celery Kale Juice

Ingredients:

1 cup of celery, chopped

1 cup of fresh kale, torn

1 cup of asparagus, trimmed

1 cup of mustard greens, torn

1 large lemon

1 large cucumber

Preparation:

Wash the celery thoroughly and cut into bite-sized pieces. Set aside.

Combine kale and mustard greens in a colander and wash under cold running water. Torn with hands and set aside.

Wash the asparagus and trim off the woody ends. Cut into small pieces and set aside.

Peel the lemon and cut lengthwise in half. Set aside.

Wash the cucumber and cut into thick slices. Set aside.

Now, process celery, kale, asparagus, mustard greens,

lemon, and cucumber in a juicer.

Transfer to serving glasses and add few ice cubes before serving.

Enjoy!

Nutritional information per serving: Kcal: 107, Protein: 10.7g, Carbs: 33g, Fats: 1.7g

38. Parsley Apple Juice

Ingredients:

2 tbsp of fresh parsley

2 large apples, cored

2 large carrots

½ cup of fresh spinach

¼ tsp of ginger, ground

1 tbsp of flaxseeds

Preparation:

Combine parsley and spinach in a large colander. Wash under cold running water. Drain and torn into small pieces. Set aside.

Wash the apples and cut in half. Remove the core and cut into bite-size pieces. Set aside. Wash the carrots and cut into thin slices. Set aside. Now, combine parsley, apples, spinach, and carrots in a juicer. Process until juiced. Transfer to serving glasses and stir in the ginger and flaxseeds. Add a few ice cubes and serve.

Nutritional information per serving: Kcal: 119, Protein: 4.3g, Carbs: 62.2g, Fats: 2.3g

39.   Zucchini Carrot Juice

Ingredients:

1 medium-sized zucchini, chunked

1 large carrot, sliced

1 large artichoke

1 red leaf lettuce, torn

1 cup of watercress, torn

3 oz of water

Preparation:

Peel the zucchini and cut in half. Scoop out the seeds and cut into chunks. Set aside. Set aside.

Wash the carrot and cut into thick slices. Set aside.

Trim off the outer leaves of the artichoke using a sharp knife. Cut into small pieces and set aside.

Combine red leaf lettuce and watercress in a colander. Wash under cold running water. Drain and torn with hands. Set aside.

Now, process zucchini, carrot, artichoke, red leaf lettuce, and watercress in a juicer. Transfer to serving glasses and stir in the water.

You can sprinkle with some fresh mint, but this is optional.

Add few ice cubes and serve immediately.

Nutritional information per serving: Kcal: 94, Protein: 9.4g, Carbs: 31.1g, Fats: 1.1g

40.   Kale Squash Juice

Ingredients:

¼ cup of fresh kale

½ yellow squash, peeled and chopped

1 medium-sized broccoli

1 large apple, cored

¼ cup of fresh spinach

4 small carrots, sliced

Preparation:

Combine kale and spinach in a large colander. Rinse under cold running water and torn into small pieces. Set aside.

Peel the squash and cut in half. Scoop out the seeds and chop into small pieces. Reserve the rest in the refrigerator.

Wash the broccoli and chop into small pieces. Set aside.

Wash the apple and cut in half. Remove the core and chop into small pieces. Set aside.

Wash and peel the carrot. Cut into small slices and set aside.

Now, combine kale, spinach, squash, broccoli, apple, and carrot in a juicer. Process until well juiced. Transfer to a serving glasses and add few ice cubes.

Serve immediately.

Nutritional information per serving: Kcal: 81, Protein: 2.3g, Carbs: 18.4g, Fats: 0.2g

41.   Strawberry Apple Juice

Ingredients:

1 cup of strawberries

1 large green apple, cored

3 large peaches, pitted

¼ tsp of cinnamon, ground

Preparation:

Wash the strawberries and remove the top stem. Chop into small pieces and fill the measuring cup. Reserve the rest in the refrigerator.

Wash the apple and cut in half. Remove the core and chop into bite-sized pieces. Set aside. Wash the peaches and cut in half. Remove the pits and chop into small pieces. Set aside.

Now, combine strawberries, apple, and peaches in a juicer. Process until juiced. Transfer to a serving glass and stir in the cinnamon. Refrigerate for 10 minutes before serving.

Nutritional information per serving: Kcal: 64, Protein: 1.2g, Carbs: 18.3g, Fats: 0.1g

42.   Blueberry Grapefruit Juice

Ingredients:

1 cup of blueberries

1 whole grapefruit, peeled

1 cup of avocado, cubed

1 small Red Delicious apple, cored

1 tsp of peppermint extract

Preparation:

Place the blueberries in a colander. Rinse well under cold running water and drain. Set aside.

Peel the grapefruit and divide into wedges. Cut each wedge in half and set aside.

Peel the avocado and cut lengthwise in half. Remove the pit and cut into small cubes. Fill the measuring cup and reserve the rest in the refrigerator.

Wash the apple and cut lengthwise in half. Remove the core and cut into bite-sized pieces. Set aside.

Now, combine blueberries, grapefruit, avocado, and apple in a juicer and process until juiced. Transfer to a serving glass and stir in the peppermint extract.

Refrigerate for 5 minutes before serving.

Nutrition information per serving: Kcal: 436, Protein: 6.4g, Carbs: 69.5g, Fats: 23.2g

43.   Lemon Papaya Juice

Ingredients:

1 large lemon, peeled and halved

1 cup of papaya, chopped

1 large green apple, cored

1 cup of cantaloupe, cubed

1 large cucumber

Preparation:

Peel the lemon and cut lengthwise in half. Set aside.

Peel the papaya and cut lengthwise in half. Scoop out the black seeds and flesh using a spoon. Cut into small chunks and fill the measuring cup. Refrigerate the rest for some other juice recipe. Set aside.

Wash the apple and remove the core. Cut into bite-sized pieces and set aside.

Cut the cantaloupe in half. Scoop out the seeds and flesh. Cut two wedges and peel them. Chop into chunks and set aside. Reserve the rest of the cantaloupe in a refrigerator.

Wash the cucumber and cut into thick slices. Set aside.

Now, process lemon, papaya, apple, cantaloupe, and cucumber in a juicer. Transfer to serving glasses and add few ice cubes before serving.

Enjoy!

Nutritional information per serving: Kcal: 245, Protein: 5.5g, Carbs: 72.8g, Fats: 1.6g

44.   Kale Apple Juice

Ingredients:

½ cup of fresh kale

1 large green apple, cored

½ cup of pomegranate seeds

¼ tsp of ginger, ground

3-4 fresh mint leaves

Preparation:

Rinse the kale thoroughly under cold running water. Drain well and torn into small pieces. Set aside. Wash the apple and cut in half. Remove the core and cut into bite-sized pieces. Set aside.

Cut the top of the pomegranate fruit using a sharp knife. Slice down to each of the white membranes inside of the fruit. Pop the seeds into a small bowl. Set aside. Now, combine kale, apple, and pomegranate seeds in a juicer and process until juiced. Transfer to serving glasses and stir in the ginger. Add few ice cubes and top with mint leaves. Add few ice cubes and serve immediately.

Nutritional information per serving: Kcal: 143, Protein: 6.2g, Carbs: 41.2g, Fats: 2.4g

45.   Orange Coconut Juice

Ingredients:

1 large orange, peeled

1 tsp of pure coconut sugar

½ cup of butternut squash, chunked

2 slices of fresh ginger

1 large red delicious apple, peeled and cored

1 large carrot, sliced

Preparation:

Peel the orange and divide into wedges. Set aside.

Peel the ginger slices and cut into small pieces. Set aside.

Combine 2 tablespoons of water and coconut sugar in a small bowl. Stir well let it stand for 5 minutes, or until sugar completely disolved.

Peel the butternut squash and remove the seeds using a spoon. Cut into small cubes and reserve the rest of the squash for some other recipe. Wrap in a plastic foil and refrigerate.

Wash the apple and remove the core. Cut into bite-sized

pieces and set aside.

Wash the carrot and cut into small slices. Set aside.

Now, process orange, ginger, butternut squash, apple, carrot, and in a juicer. Transfer to serving glasses and stir in the coconut mixture.

Add few ice cubes and serve immediately.

Nutritional information per serving: Kcal: 314, Protein: 5.3g, Carbs: 61g, Fats: 1.2g

46.   Italian Vegetable Juice

Ingredients:

3 large cucumbers

1 large bell pepper, seeded

2 large tomatoes, halved

2 garlic cloves, peeled

1 large lime, peeled

¼ cup of fresh cilantro

Preparation:

Wash the cucumber and chop into thin slices. Set aside.

Wash the bell pepper and cut in half. Remove the seeds and chop into small pieces. Set aside.

Wash the tomatoes and chop into small pieces. Make sure to reserve the tomato juice while cutting. Set aside.

Peel the lime and cut in half. Set aside.

Wash the cilantro and chop into small pieces. Set aside.

Now, combine cucumber, bell pepper, tomatoes, lime, and cilantro in a juicer. Process until juiced. Transfer to a serving glass and serve immediately.

Nutritional information per serving: Kcal: 109, Protein: 6.4g, Carbs: 38.5g, Fats: 1.2g

47.   Carrot Cucumber Juice

Ingredients:

1 large carrot

1 large cucumber

1 cup of butternut squash, chopped

1 large guava

1 large orange

1 tbsp of honey

Preparation:

Wash the carrot and cut into thin slices. Set aside.

Peel the cucumber and cut into thin slices. Set aside.

Peel the butternut squash and remove the seeds using a spoon. Cut into small cubes and reserve the rest of the squash for some other recipe. Wrap in a plastic foil and refrigerate.

Peel the guava and cut into chunks. Set aside.

Now, combine, carrot, cucumber, butternut squash, guava, and orange in a juicer and process until juiced.

Transfer to serving glasses and stir in the honey.

Add some ice and serve immediately.

Nutritional information per serving: Kcal: 266, Protein: 7.2g, Carbs: 80.7g, Fats: 1.4g

48. Lemon Banana Juice

Ingredients:

1 whole lemon, peeled

1 large banana, chunked

1 cup of strawberries, chopped

1 cup of pineapple, chunked

1 tbsp of fresh mint, finely chopped

Preparation:

Peel the lemon and cut lengthwise in half. Set aside.

Peel the banana and cut into small chunks. Set aside.

Wash the strawberries and remove the stems. Chop into small pieces and fill the measuring cup. Reserve the rest in the refrigerator.

Cut the top of the pineapple using a sharp paring knife. Gently remove all hard skin and slice it into thin slices. Fill the measuring cup and reserve the rest for later.

Now, combine lemon, banana, strawberries, and pineapple in a juicer. Process until juiced. Transfer to a serving glass and stir in the mint.

Add few ice cubes and serve immediately.

Nutrition information per serving: Kcal: 224, Protein: 4.1g, Carbs: 69.4g, Fats: 1.3g

49.   Pepper Basil Juice

Ingredients:

2 large red bell peppers, chopped

1 cup of fresh basil, torn

3 large beets, trimmed

1 large lime, peeled and halved

1 cup of red leaf lettuce, torn

 1 large cucumber

Preparation:

Wash the red bell peppers and cut in half. Remove the seeds and roughly chop it. Set aside.

Wash the beets and trim off the green parts. Cut into small pieces and set aside.

Peel the lime and cut lengthwise in half. Set aside.

Combine basila and red leaf lettuce in a large colander and wash thoroughly under cold running water. Drain and torn into small pieces. Set aside.

Wash the cucumber and cut into thin slices. Set aside.

Now, process red bell peppers, basil, beets, lime, red leaf lettuce, and cucumber in a juicer. Transfer to serving glasses and add few ice cubes.

Serve immediately.

Nutritional information per serving: Kcal: 208, Protein: 10.5g, Carbs: 59.2g, Fats: 1.9g

50.   Basil Lime Juice

Ingredients:

½ cup of fresh basil

1 large lime, peeled

½ cup of Swiss chard

2 large green apples, cored

¼ cup of fresh mint

Preparation:

Combine basil, Swiss chard, and mint in a large colander and rinse under cold running water. Drain and torn into small pieces. Set aside.

Peel the lime and cut lengthwise in half. Set aside.

Wash the apples and cut in half. Remove the core and cut into bite-sized pieces. Set aside. Now, combine basil, Swiss chard, mint, lime, and apples in a juicer. Process until well juiced. Transfer to serving glasses and add few ice cubes or refrigerate until use.

Nutritional information per serving: Kcal: 114, Protein: 2.3g, Carbs: 30.4g, Fats: 0.2g

51.   Radish Beet Juice

Ingredients:

3 large radishes, chopped

2 cups of beet greens, torn

2 large leeks, chopped

1 cup of collard greens, torn

1 large cucumber

½ tsp of Himalayan salt

¼ tsp of Cayenne pepper, ground

3 oz of water

Preparation:

Wash the radishes and trim off the green parts. Cut in half and set aside.

Combine beet greens and collard greens in a colander. Wash thoroughly under cold running water. Drain and set aside.

Wash the leeks and chop into small pieces. Set aside.

Wash the cucumber and cut into thick slices. Set aside-

Now, combine radishes, beet greens, leeks, collard greens, and cucumber in a juicer and process until juiced.

Transfer to serving glasses and stir in the salt, Cayenne pepper, and water.

Refrigerate for 10 minutes before serving.

Enjoy!

Nutritional information per serving: Kcal: 148, Protein: 7.6g, Carbs: 42.3g, Fats: 1.2g

52.   Carrot Watercress Juice

Ingredients:

2 large carrots, sliced

½ cup of watercress, torn

1 cup of pineapple, chunked

1 large lemon, peeled

¼ tsp of fresh ginger root, ground

Preparation:

Wash and peel the carrots. Cut into thin slices and set aside.

Rinse the watercress under cold running water. Drain well and torn into small pieces. Fill the measuring cup and reserve the rest for later.

Cut the top of a pineapple and peel it using a sharp knife. Cut into small chunks and fill the measuring cup. Reserve the rest of the pineapple in a refrigerator.

Peel the lemon and cut lengthwise in half. Set aside.

Now, combine carrots, watercress, pineapple, and lemon in a juicer. Process until juiced. Transfer to a serving glass and stir in the ginger.

Add some ice and serve.

Nutritional information per serving: Kcal: 101, Protein: 3.1g, Carbs: 34.2g, Fats: 1.1g

53.   Pineapple Orange Juice

Ingredients:

1 cup of pineapple chunks

1 large orange, peeled and wedged

1 cup of avocado, cubed

1 large cucumber, sliced

2 oz of water

Preparation:

Cut the top of a pineapple and peel it using a sharp knife. Cut into small chunks. Reserve the rest of the pineapple in a refrigerator.

Peel the orange and divide into wedges. Set aside.

Peel the avocado and cut in half. Remove the pit and cut into small cubes. Fill the measuring cup and reserve the rest in the refrigerator.

Wash the cucumber and cut into thick slices. Set aside.

Now, combine pineapple, orange, avocado, and cucumber in a juicer and process until juiced.

Transfer to serving glasses and stir in the water. Add few

ice cubes and serve immediately.

Nutritional information per serving: Kcal: 375, Protein: 7.5g, Carbs: 66.6g, Fats: 22.15g

54.   Tomato Mustard Green Juice

Ingredients:

1 medium-sized Roma tomato, chopped

1 cup of mustard greens, torn

2 cups of Romaine lettuce, chopped

1 cup of parsley, torn

1 whole cucumber, sliced

¼ tsp of turmeric, ground

¼ tsp of salt

Preparation:

Wash the tomato and place in a bowl. Chop into bite-sized pieces and reserve the tomato juice while cutting. Set aside.

Combine mustard greens, lettuce, and parsley in a large colander. Rinse well and drain. Torn into small pieces and set aside.

Wash the cucumber and cut into thin slices. Set aside.

Now, combine tomato, mustard greens, lettuce, parsley, and cucumber in a juicer and process until juiced. Transfer to a serving glass and stir in the turmeric, salt, and reserved tomato juice.

Refrigerate for 5 minutes before serving.

Enjoy!

Nutrition information per serving: Kcal: 85, Protein: 7.6g, Carbs: 25.3g, Fats: 1.6g

55.   Peach Pomegranate Juice

Ingredients:

2 large peaches, pitted

1 cup of pomegranate seeds

5 large plums, pitted

1 large carrot

Preparation:

Wash the plums and peaches and cut in half. Remove the pits and set aside.

Cut the top of the pomegranate fruit using a sharp knife. Slice down to each of the white membranes inside of the fruit. Pop the seeds into a small bowl. Set aside.

Wash the carrot and cut into small pieces. Set aside.

Now, combine plums, peaches, pomegranate seeds, and carrot in a juicer and process until juiced.

Transfer to serving glasses and refrigerate for 10 minutes before serving.

Nutritional information per serving: Kcal: 326, Protein: 7.6g, Carbs: 94.2g, Fats: 3.1g

56.   Beet Lime Juice

Ingredients:

1 small cauliflower head, chopped

2 large beets, trimmed

1 large lime, peeled and halved

2 large radishes, chopped

¼ tsp of Himalayan salt

3 oz of water

Preparation:

Wash the beets and radishes. Trim off the green parts and cut into bite-sized pieces. Set aside. Peel the lime and cut lengthwise in half. Set aside.

Trim off the outer leaves of cauliflower. Wash it and cut into small pieces. Set aside. Now, combine beets, lime, cauliflower, and radishes in a juicer. Transfer to serving glasses and stir in the salt and water.

Add some ice cubes and serve immediately.

Nutritional information per serving: Kcal: 135, Protein: 9.3g, Carbs: 41g, Fats: 1.2g

57.   Melon Apple Juice

Ingredients:

1 large wedge of honeydew melon

1 small Grany Smith's apple, cored

2 cups of blueberries

1 oz of coconut water

1 tsp of vanilla extract

1 tbsp of mint, finely chopped

Preparation:

Cut melon lengthwise in half. Scoop out the seeds and then wash. Cut one large wedge and peel it. Cut into small cubes and set aside.

Wash the apple and cut lengthwise in half. Remove the core and cut into bite-sized pieces. Set aside.

Place the blueberries in a large colander. Rinse well under cold running water and drain. Set aside.

Now, combine honeydew melon, apple, and blueberries in a juicer. Process until juiced.

Transfer to a serving glass and stir in the coconut water,

vanilla extract, and mint. Add some crushed ice and serve immediately.

Nutrition information per serving: Kcal: 263, Protein: 3.7g, Carbs: 77.1g, Fats: 1.5g

58.   Grapefruit Rosemary Juice

Ingredients:

3 large grapefruits, peeled

3 large oranges, peeled

1 large lemon, peeled

½ tsp of fresh rosemary

Preparation:

Peel the grapefruit and oranges. Cut into bite-sized pieces. Set aside.

Peel the lemon and cut lengthwise in half. Set aside.

Combine all ingredients in a juicer and process until juiced. Transfer to serving glasses and add few ice cubes.

Sprinkle with fresh rosemary and serve immediately!

Nutritional information per serving: Kcal: 140, Protein: 3.4g, Carbs: 37.6g, Fats: 0.1g

59.   Carrot Lemon Juice

Ingredients:

3 large carrots

1 large lemon, peeled

1 cup of green beans

1 cup of fresh kale, torn

1 large cucumber

1 tbsp of honey, raw

Preparation:

Wash the carrots and cut into thick slices. Set aside.

Peel the lemon and cut lengthwise in half. Set aside.

Wash the kale thoroughly under cold running water. Drain and set aside.

Wash the green beans and place them in a medium pot. Add water enough to cover and soak for at least 2 hours. Set aside.

Now, process carrots, lemon, green beans, kale, and cucumber in a juicer.

Transfer to serving glasses and stir in the honey. Refrigerate for 5 minutes and serve.

Enjoy!

Nutritional information per serving: Kcal: 239, Protein: 9.4g, Carbs: 50g, Fats: 1.8g

60.   Lime Beet Juice

Ingredients:

2 large limes, peeled

1 cup of beet greens, torn

2 large cucumbers, peeled

1 cup of kale, chopped

1 cup of parsley, chopped

1 tbsp of agave syrup

½ cup of pure coconut water, unsweetened

Preparation:

Peel the limes and cut into quarters and add to the bowl.

Wash the beet greens and torn into a bowl with other ingredients.

Wash the cucumbers and cut into thick slices. Place them in a medium bowl and set aside.

Combine parsley and kale in a colander and wash with cold running water. Roughly chop it and add to the bowl.

Now, process limes, beet greens, cucumber, kale, and

parsley in a juicer. Transfer to serving glasses and stir in the agave syrup and coconut water.

Add some ice and serve immediately.

Nutritional information per serving: Kcal: 139, Protein: 10.6g, Carbs: 42.2g, Fats: 1.9g

61.　　Apple Orange Juice

Ingredients:

1 medium-sized red apple, cored

1 large orange, peeled

2 large peaches, chopped

1 ginger root knob, 1-inch

2 oz of water

Preparation:

Wash the apple and remove the core. Cut into bite-sized pieces and set aside.

Peel the orange and divide into wedges. Set aside.

Wash the peaches and cut in half. Remove the pits and cut into small pieces. Set aside. Peel the ginger root knob and set aside.

Now, process apple, orange, peaches, and ginger in a juicer. Transfer to serving glasses and stir in the water. Add some ice or refrigerate before serving.

Nutritional information per serving: Kcal: 294, Protein: 5.6g, Carbs: 85.8g, Fats: 1.5g

62.   Asparagus Broccoli Juice

Ingredients:

4 medium-sized asparagus spears, trimmed

1 large broccoli

1 large green apple, cored

3 large celery stalks

A handful of fresh parsley

Preparation:

Wash the asparagus and trim off the woody ends. Cut into small pieces and set aside.

Wash the celery stalks and broccoli. Chop into small pieces. Set aside.

Wash the apple and remove the core. Cut into bite-sized pieces and set aside.

Wash the parsley and finely chop it. Place it in a small bowl and add olive oil. Let it stand for 5 minutes.

Now, process asparagus, broccoli, apple, and celery in a juicer. Transfer to serving glasses and stir in the parsley and oil. You can sprinkle with some salt to taste if you like, but this is optional.

Serve immediately.

Nutritional information per serving: Kcal: 134, Protein: 7.3g, Carbs: 45.9g, Fats: 1.7g

63.　Mango Apple Juice

Ingredients:

1 cup of mango chunks

1 medium-sized green apple, cored

1 cup of cranberries

1 large honeydew melon wedge, chopped

1 cup of fresh mint

½ cup of hot water

Preparation:

Peel the mango and cut into chunks. Set aside.

Wash the apple and remove the core. Cut into bite-sized pieces and set aside.

Place the cranberries in a colander and wash under cold running water. Drain and set aside.

Cut the honeydew melon lengthwise in half. Scoop out the seeds using a spoon. Cut the large wedges and peel them. Cut into small chunks and place in a bowl. Wrap the rest of the melon in a plastic foil and refrigerate.

Combine mint with hot water and let it stand for 5 minutes.

Now, process mango, apple, cranberries, honeydew melon, and mint in a juicer. Transfer to serving glasses and add water from the soaked mint. Refrigerate for 5 minutes before serving.

Nutritional information per serving: Kcal: 261, Protein: 4.3g, Carbs: 79.1g, Fats: 1.5g

64. Blueberry Basil Juice

Ingredients:

1 cup of blackberries

1 cup of blueberries

1 cup of fresh basil

1 large beet, trimmed

2 oz of coconut water

Preparation:

Combine blackberries and blueberries in a colander and wash under cold running water. Set aside.

Wash the basil thoroughly and roughly chop it using hands.

Wash the beet and trim off the green ends. Chop into small pieces and set aside.

Now, combine blueberries, basil, blackberries, and beet in a juicer and process until juiced. Transfer to serving glasses and stir in the coconut water.

Add some ice and serve immediately.

Nutritional information per serving: Kcal: 142, Protein: 5.2g, Carbs: 44.8g, Fats: 1.5g

65.   Watercress Basil Juice

Ingredients:

1 cup of watercress, torn

1 cup of basil, torn

5 plum tomatoes, halved

1 large green bell pepper

1 large cucumber

A handful of spinach

Preparation:

Combine watercress, basil, and spinach in a colander. Wash thoroughly under cold running water. Drain and torn with hands. Set aside.

Wash the plum tomatoes and place them in a bowl. Cut in half and reserve the juice while cutting. Set aside.

Wash the green bell pepper and cut in half. Remove the seeds and chop into small pieces. Set aside.

Wash the cucumber and cut into thick slices. Set aside.

Now, process watercress, basil, plum tomatoes, spinach, green bell pepper, and cucumber in a juicer. Transfer to serving glasses and stir in the salt and water.

Add some ice and serve.

Nutritional information per serving: Kcal: 112, Protein: 8.5g, Carbs: 32.7g, Fats: 1.5g

66.   Orange Pumpkin Juice

Ingredients:

1 large orange, peeled

¼ tsp of pumpkin pie spice

2 large carrots

1 small sweet potato, peeled

2 medium-sized green apples, cored

Preparation:

Peel the orange and divide into wedges. Cut each wedge in half and set aside.

Wash the carrots and chop into small pieces.

Combine all ingredients except pumpkin pie spice in a juicer and process until juiced.

Transfer the juice to serving glasses and add few ice cubes.

Sprinkle with some pumpkin pie spice and serve.

Nutritional information per serving: Kcal: 147, Protein: 2.1g, Carbs: 35.4g, Fats: 0.1g

ADDITIONAL TITLES FROM THIS AUTHOR

70 Effective Meal Recipes to Prevent and Solve Being Overweight: Burn Fat Fast by Using Proper Dieting and Smart Nutrition

By

Joe Correa CSN

48 Acne Solving Meal Recipes: The Fast and Natural Path to Fixing Your Acne Problems in Less Than 10 Days!

By

Joe Correa CSN

41 Alzheimer's Preventing Meal Recipes: Reduce or Eliminate Your Alzheimer's Condition in 30 Days or Less!

By

Joe Correa CSN

70 Effective Breast Cancer Meal Recipes: Prevent and Fight Breast Cancer with Smart Nutrition and Powerful Foods

By

Joe Correa CSN

www.ingramcontent.com/pod-product-compliance
Lightning Source LLC
Chambersburg PA
CBHW030243030426
42336CB00009B/230